Clinical Pocket Manual™

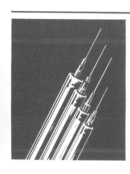

Medications and I.V.s

NURSING87 BOOKS™
SPRINGHOUSE CORPORATION
SPRINGHOUSE, PENNSYLVANIA

Clinical Pocket Manual™ Series

PROGRAM DIRECTOR
Jean Robinson

ART DIRECTOR
John Hubbard

EDITORS
Katherine W. Carey
Kathy E. Goldberg

CLINICAL EDITORS
Joan E. Mason, RN, EdM
Diane Schweisguth, RN, BSN

PROJECT COORDINATOR
Aline S. Miller

EDITORIAL SERVICES
MANAGER
David R. Moreau

DESIGNER
Maria Errico

PRODUCTION COORDINATOR
Maureen B. Carmichael

The clinical procedures described and recommended in this publication are based on research and consultation with medical and nursing authorities. To the best of our knowledge, these procedures reflect currently accepted clinical practice; nevertheless, they can't be considered absolute and universal recommendations. For individual application, treatment recommendations must be considered in light of the patient's clinical condition and, before administration of new or infrequently used drugs, in light of latest package-insert information. The authors and the publisher disclaim responsibility for any adverse effects resulting directly or indirectly from the suggested procedures, from any undetected errors, or from the reader's misunderstanding of the text.

Material in this book was adapted from the following series: Nurse's Reference Library, Nursing Photobook, New Nursing Skillbook, Nursing Now, and Nurse's Clinical Library.

Library of Congress Cataloging-in-Publication Data

Medications and I.V.s.

(Clinical pocket manual)
"Nursing87 books."
Includes index.
1. Chemotherapy—Handbooks, manuals, etc.
2. Intravenous therapy—Handbooks, manuals, etc.
3. Nursing—Handbooks, manuals, etc.
I. Springhouse Corporation.   II. Title: Medications and IVs.   III. Series. [DNLM: 1. Drug Therapy—handbooks. 2. Drug Therapy—nurses' instruction.
3. Fluid Therapy—handbooks. 4. Fluid Therapy—nurses' instruction. 5. Infusions, Parenteral—handbooks. 6. Infusions, Parenteral—nurses' instruction. WB 39 M4895]
RM262.M394   1987   615'.63   86-30096
ISBN 0-87434-013-6

CONTENTS

1 Medication and I.V. Basics
Administration Guidelines 1-11; Calculations 12-18; I.V. Procedures 19-22

23 Oral and Dermatomucosal Medications
Oral Medications 23-29; Sublingual and Buccal Medications 30; Tube Medication Administration 31-35; Rectal Medications 36-39; Vaginal Medications 40; Topical Medications 41-46; Eye Medications 47-50; Ear Medications 51-52; Nasal Medications 53-55; Mouth and Throat Medications 56; Inhalation Medications 57-62; Endotracheal Medication Administration 63

64 Parenteral Medications
Administration Guidelines 64-70; Intradermal Injections 71-73; Subcutaneous Injections 74-79; I.M. Injections 80-86; I.V. Injections 87-101; Intraarterial Injections 102-103; Intrathecal Injections 104; Special Devices 105

106 I.V. Therapy
Administration Guidelines 106-120; Fluids and Fluid Therapy 121-122; I.V. Hyperalimentation 123-128; Blood and Blood Products 129-137

138 Special Considerations
Pediatric Medication Administration 138-140; Medications and the Elderly Patient 141-144; Special Problems 145-149; I.V. Controllers and Pumps 150-153; Drug Abuse and Toxicity 154-160; Drug Interactions 161-183

Nursing87 Books™

CLINICAL POCKET MANUAL™ SERIES

Diagnostic Tests
Emergency Care
Fluids and Electrolytes
Signs and Symptoms
Cardiovascular Care
Respiratory Care
Critical Care
Neurologic Care
Surgical Care
Medications and I.V.s
Ob/Gyn Care
Pediatric Care

NURSING NOW™ SERIES

Shock
Hypertension
Drug Interactions
Cardiac Crises
Respiratory Emergencies
Pain

NURSE'S CLINICAL LIBRARY®

Cardiovascular Disorders
Respiratory Disorders
Endocrine Disorders
Neurologic Disorders
Renal and Urologic Disorders
Gastrointestinal Disorders
Neoplastic Disorders
Immune Disorders

NURSE'S REFERENCE LIBRARY®

Diseases	Definitions
Diagnostics	Practices
Drugs	Emergencies
Assessment	Signs & Symptoms
Procedures	Patient Teaching

NURSING PHOTOBOOK™ SERIES

Providing Respiratory Care
Managing I.V. Therapy
Dealing with Emergencies
Giving Medications
Assessing Your Patients
Using Monitors
Providing Early Mobility
Giving Cardiac Care
Performing GI Procedures
Implementing Urologic Procedures
Controlling Infection
Ensuring Intensive Care
Coping with Neurologic Disorders
Caring for Surgical Patients
Working with Orthopedic Patients
Nursing Pediatric Patients
Helping Geriatric Patients
Attending Ob/Gyn Patients
Aiding Ambulatory Patients
Carrying Out Special Procedures

NURSE REVIEW™ SERIES

Cardiac Problems
Respiratory Problems
Gastrointestinal Problems
Neurologic Problems
Vascular Problems
Genitourinary Problems
Endocrine Problems
Musculoskeletal Problems

Nursing87 DRUG HANDBOOK™

Observing the Five Rights

Before you give *any* medication, compare the doctor's order with the order written on your patient's medication card or Kardex. To do this correctly and efficiently, use the system known as the Five Rights. Ask yourself the questions listed below.

If you find any discrepancy—no matter how small—withhold the medication until you can check with the doctor or pharmacist. Doing so will prevent errors and ensure safe administration.

- Right name: Is the patient's *name* the same?
- Right drug: Is the ordered *drug* the same?
- Right dose: Is the ordered *dose* the same?
- Right route: Is the ordered *route* the same?
- Right time and frequency: Is the *time and frequency* of administration the same?

Verbal Medication Orders

Never accept a verbal medication order from anyone, except in an extreme emergency. If such an emergency occurs, write the order on the patient's chart so you can refer to it easily. Then have the doctor countersign it as soon as possible.

MEDICATION AND I.V. BASICS

Administering Medications: Important Implications

Follow these general guidelines when administering medications to adults:

• Never administer medication (not even a placebo) without a doctor's orders.

• Carry out verbal orders only in emergencies, and then with extreme care to ensure accuracy. Such orders must follow established hospital policy.

• Avoid using the patient's own medications. Use them only if the doctor writes an appropriate order on the chart and the pharmacy can't obtain the drugs. All such drugs must first be identified by a pharmacist. If they can't be identified, don't use them.

• Know why every drug you administer has been prescribed, its usual dose range, its expected action, and its possible adverse effects. To properly assess the effects a medication may have on your patient's condition, ask yourself these questions:

—Is the prescribed medication appropriate for the patient's present or preexisting condition?

—Is the dose within safe limits?

—Is the ordered route compatible with the patient's condition?

—Is the medication compatible with other medications the patient's taking?

—What foods or other medications will affect its absorption?

—What's the medication's expected effect?

—What adverse effects could the medication cause?

• Remember that names of different drugs may have similar spellings. Check each carefully. Never identify an item merely by its container, appearance, or customary shelf location. Check labels for expiration date. If the bottle has no label, return it to the pharmacy.

• Always wash your hands thoroughly before preparing or administering medication.

• Only the nurse who prepares a medication should administer it.

• When preparing medications, guard against interruptions. If you have any doubt about a dose calculation, physical appearance, or drug name, ask the pharmacist, check a proper drug reference, or double-check calculations with another nurse.

Continued

Administering Medications: Important Implications
Continued

- Don't hold tablets or capsules in your hands.
- Administer medications as close as possible (within hospital requirements) to the time officially prescribed.
- Before administering a drug, read the label three times (when taking the drug container from the shelf or cart bin, when preparing the dose, and when returning the drug to storage).
- Don't give medication that's discolored or in which a precipitate has formed unless the manufacturer's instructions indicate that doing so won't cause harm.
- Always tightly replace the cap on any medication bottle you open. Never leave a single capsule of a desiccant in a bottle—discard it to avoid giving it to a patient inadvertently. Don't leave any medication bottles lying about.
- Never leave medications at a patient's bedside except on doctor's orders—unless the patient's permitted to administer to himself.

- Check the patient's armband for proper identification; then address him by name or ask the patient his name. Don't ask, "Are you Mr. Wilson?" If the patient's not alert, he may answer yes without realizing what he's saying.
- Always recheck when a patient expresses doubt or concern about the medication you're going to give him. Make sure you're giving the *right dose* of the *right medication* to the *right patient* at the *right time* by the *right route*.
- Check the patient's allergy history. If the prescribed medication contains a component that the patient's allergic to, withhold the drug until you've consulted the doctor. If the Kardex doesn't include allergy information, don't assume the patient has no allergies. Question the patient and/or a family member before giving any new medication.
- If the patient refuses to take his medication, try to find out why.
- When administering drugs p.r.n., always determine that enough time has passed since the last dose.

Does Your Patient Have an Allergy?

You know how important it is to have accurate allergy information when you're administering a medication. But do you always give that information the attention it deserves? You can endanger a patient's life if you administer a medication to which he's allergic. Avoid a serious error like this by following these precautions:

• Anytime you receive a new medication order for your patient, familiarize yourself with the medication's components before administering it.

Take, for example, the nurse who administers Percodan* to a patient with an aspirin allergy. Percodan, as you probably know, contains aspirin. Looking up the medication *before* she administered it could have prevented the patient from developing anaphylactic shock.

• Before giving a patient any medication, check his Kardex in the appropriate space for allergy information.

• If no allergy information is listed on the Kardex, don't assume that the patient has no allergies. Question the patient and his family. Then, if he *does* have an allergy, add the information to his Kardex. If the patient has never received a medication such as penicillin, but several members of his family are allergic to it, assume that he's allergic to penicillin also. Get an order for a substitute antibiotic. If he has no allergies, write: "None known."

*Available in the United States and Canada

MEDICATION AND I.V. BASICS

How to Cope with Unexpected Problems

If you've ever given medications, you know unexpected problems can disrupt normal routine. Study this chart for tips on how to deal with them.

PROBLEM	POSSIBLE EXPLANATIONS	INTERVENTIONS
You can't find the ordered medication in the patient's medication drawer.	• An error was detected on the Kardex, so the order was withheld until the doctor could be notified. • The medication was replaced with a generic substitute. • The pharmacy hasn't dispensed the medication yet. • The medication was placed in someone else's bin.	• Go to the order sheet and double-check your information. If it's correct, ask the pharmacy about the medication order. If the order is still unfilled or was filled (and the medication misplaced), chart the reason why you didn't give the medication. If the medication was replaced with a generic substitute, give that substitute to the patient.
You find a medication in the patient's medication drawer, but no order is written on the Kardex.	• The ordered medication was never transcribed on the Kardex. • The medication was meant for a patient with the same name on another unit. • The medication was discontinued but not removed from the drawer.	• Do not administer the medication until you can go to the order sheet and double-check your information. Then, if it checks out, transcribe the order on the Kardex, and administer the medication. If there's no order for the medication, return it to the pharmacy with an explanation.

Continued

How to Cope with Unexpected Problems
Continued

PROBLEM	POSSIBLE EXPLANATIONS	INTERVENTIONS
You notice that the medication does not look the same as it usually does; for example, it's cloudy or a different color.	• The medication has deteriorated. • The hospital is buying medication in a new generic form. • The wrong medication was placed in the container.	• In such a case, withhold the medication until you can check with the pharmacist. Then, if you don't administer it, chart the reason why.
You discover that the medication container isn't labeled.	• The label has fallen off.	• Withhold the medication. Then return the container for relabeling. Document why the medication wasn't administered.
Your patient tells you he never received medication like this before.	• The medication is wrong and was ordered by mistake. • The medication is a new order. • The patient is confused.	• Withhold the medication. Then, if the medication wasn't ordered, consult with the doctor, and document why you withheld it. If it was ordered, tell your patient the name of the medication and why it was prescribed.

Drugs and the Law

Legally, a *drug* is any substance listed in an official state, Canadian provincial, or national formulary. It may also be any substance (other than food) "intended to affect the structure or any function of the body...(or) for use in the diagnosis, cure, mitigation, treatment, or prevention of disease" (N.Y. Educ. Law).

A *prescription drug* is any drug restricted from regular commercial purchase and sale because a state, provincial, or national government has determined that it is, or might be, unsafe unless used under a qualified medical practitioner's supervision.

Drug laws
Two federal laws mainly govern the use of drugs in the United States: the Comprehensive Drug Abuse Prevention and Control Act (incorporating the Controlled Substances Act) and the Food, Drug, and Cosmetic Act.

The main laws affecting the distribution of drugs are the pharmacy practice acts. These laws give pharmacists (and sometimes doctors, in Canada) the *sole legal authority* to prepare, compound, preserve, and dispense drugs. *Dispense* refers to taking a drug from the pharmacy supply and giving or selling it to another person. This contrasts with *administering* drugs—actually getting the drug into the patient. Your nurse practice act is the law that most directly affects how you administer drugs.

In many states, if a nurse prescribes a drug, she's practicing medicine without a license; if she goes into the pharmacy or drug supply cabinet, measures out doses of a drug, and puts the powder into capsules, she's practicing pharmacy without a license. For either action, she can be prosecuted or lose her license (or both), even if no one is harmed by what she does.

Continued

Drugs and the Law
Continued

Your liability for dispensing drugs

In rare instances, adequate patient care may require that you give a certain drug that isn't available on the floor. Normally, of course, you'd call the hospital pharmacist and ask that the drug be sent. But what can you do if you're working on the night or weekend shift and no pharmacist is available?

In this situation, a nurse can't escape liability if she dispenses the drug herself and a lawsuit results. Some hospitals and nursing homes have written policies that permit the charge nurse under special circumstances to go into the pharmacy and dispense an emergency dose of a drug. But whether the institution has a written policy or not, a nurse who dispenses drugs is doing so unlawfully—unless her state's pharmacy practice act specifically authorizes her to do so. If she makes an error in dispensing the drug and the patient later sues, the fact that she was practicing as an unlicensed pharmacist can be used as evidence against her.

Your responsibility for knowing about drugs

Once you have your nursing license, you're expected—by law—to know about any drug you administer. This means you're expected to know a drug's safe dosage limits, toxicity, side effects, potential adverse reactions, and indications and contraindications for use.

Increasingly, judges and juries also expect nurses to know the appropriate observation intervals for a patient receiving any medication. And they expect you to know this even if the doctor doesn't know, or if he doesn't write an order stating how often to check on the newly medicated patient.

Continued

Drugs and the Law
Continued

MEDICATION AND I.V.
BASICS

When you must refuse to administer a drug

All nurses have the legal right not to administer drugs they think will harm patients.

You may choose to exercise this right in a variety of situations:

• when you think the dose prescribed is too high

• when you think the drug is contraindicated because of possible dangerous interactions with other drugs or with nondrugs such as alcohol

• when you think the patient's physical condition contraindicates using the drug.

In limited circumstances, you may also legally refuse to administer a drug on grounds of conscience.

When you refuse to carry out a drug order, be sure you do the following:

• Notify your immediate supervisor so she can make alternative arrangements.

• Notify the prescribing doctor if your supervisor hasn't done this already.

• If your employer requires it, document that the drug wasn't given, and explain why.

Protecting yourself from liability

If you make an error in giving a drug, or if your patient reacts negatively to a properly administered drug, protect yourself by documenting the incident thoroughly.

Some documentation belongs in the patient's chart. Besides normal drug-charting information, include information on the patient's reaction and any medical or nursing interventions taken to minimize harm to the patient.

Other documentation should be confined to the incident report. Here, identify what happened, the names and functions of all personnel involved, and what actions were taken to protect the patient after the error was discovered.

Administering Controlled Drugs: Taking the Proper Precautions

In the United States and Canada, government agencies regulate certain drugs that have a high potential for abuse. In the United States, the Food and Drug Administration divides these controlled substances into five groups, Schedules I to V. In Canada, the Health Protection Branch groups all controlled drugs into one group, Schedule G. The chart below lists the drugs in each category.

You'll never administer Schedule I drugs; they have the highest potential for abuse and aren't accepted for any medical use. But you you may administer Schedule II to V drugs, or Schedule G drugs in Canada.

Remember that all these drugs are potentially habit-forming and addictive. Before administering them, take these precautions:
- Check your hospital's policy for special procedures.
- Sign out, on the narcotics form, any drugs you remove from the narcotics cabinet.
- Follow the proper disposal procedures if any part of the drug remains after use.
- Never leave any drugs lying on the counter.
- Relock the narcotics cabinet after you've removed the drugs you need.

SCHEDULE	EXAMPLES
In the United States:	
I: No accepted medical use in the United States, with high potential for abuse	heroin, lysergic acid diethylamide (LSD), mescaline, peyote, and psilocybin
II: High potential for abuse, with severe psychological or physical dependence possible	amobarbital, amphetamine, cocaine, codeine, hydromorphone, meperidine, methadone, methamphetamine, methaqualone, methylphenidate, morphine, opium, oxycodone, oxymorphone, pen-

Continued

MEDICATION AND I.V.
BASICS

Administering Controlled Drugs: Taking the Proper Precautions
Continued

SCHEDULE	EXAMPLES
II—*continued*	tobarbital, phenmetrazine, secobarbital, and tetrahydrocannabinol (THC) and derivatives
III: Less abuse potential than drugs in Schedule II	barbituric acid derivatives (except those listed in another schedule), benzphetamine, chlorphentermine, glutethimide, mazindol, methyprylon, paregoric, and phendimetrazine
IV: Less abuse potential than drugs in Schedule III	barbital, benzodiazepine derivatives, chloral hydrate, diethylpropion, ethchlorvynol, ethinamate, fenfluramine, meprobamate, methohexital, phenobarbital, paraldehyde, and phentermine
V: Less abuse potential than drugs in Schedule IV	diphenoxylate compound and expectorants with codeine
In Canada:	
G	all salts and derivatives of the following: amphetamine, barbituric acid, benzphetamine, butorphanol, chlorphentermine, diethylpropion, methamphetamine, methaqualone, methylphenidate, pentazocine, phendimetrazine, phenmetrazine, and phentermine

Frequently Used Equivalents in the Metric System

The metric system—also called the decimal system—is used most commonly because of its accuracy. Any changes of units of measure can be made by multiplying or dividing by 10.

Metric Weight

1 gram	= 0.001 kilogram (kg or Kg)
(g, gm, Gm)	= 0.01 hectogram (hg or Hg)
	= 0.1 dekagram (dag or Dg)
	= 10 decigrams (dg)
	= 100 centigrams (cg)
	= 1,000 milligrams (mg)

Metric Volume

1 liter (L or l)	= 0.001 kiloliter (kl or Kl)
	= 0.01 hectoliter (hl or Hl)
	= 0.1 dekaliter (dal or Dl)
	= 10 deciliters (dl)
	= 100 centiliters (cl)
	= 1,000 milliliters (ml)*

*1 ml = 1 cubic centimeter (cc); however, ml is the preferred measurement term today.

Metric Weight and Volume Scale

Metric volume	kl	hl	dal	L	dl	cl	ml
Metric weight	kg	hg	dag	g	dg	cg	mg

2.35kg =   7.543 g =

23.5 hg =   75.43 dg =

235 dag =   754.3 cg =

2,350 g   7,543 mg

This graph shows the relationship between units of weight and units of volume in the metric system.

Frequently Used Equivalents in the Apothecary System

The apothecary system, an old English method of measurement, is being replaced by the metric system. However, it is still used by some doctors and hospital staffs.

The terms *fluidram* and *fluidounce* are usually shortened to *dram* and *ounce,* with the understanding that drugs in liquid form are measured by volume and those in solid form by weight. When symbols are used, quantity is expressed in small Roman numerals placed after the symbol; for example, ii. If a fraction of a measure is ordered, a symbol is not used; instead, the amount is written out with the fraction first; for example, ⅕ ounce. An exception to this is one half, which has its own symbol (ss̄). Thus an order for one half ounce can be written as ss̄ or ½ ounce.

Apothecary Weight	*Apothecary Volume*
20 grains (gr) = 1 scruple	60 minims* = 1 fluidram
3 scruples = 1 dram	8 fluidrams = 1 fluidounce
8 drams = 1 ounce	16 fluidounces = 1 pint (pt)
12 ounces = 1 pound (lb)	2 pints = 1 quart (qt)
	4 quarts = 1 gallon (gal)

*A minim is *almost equal* to a drop. When a drug is prescribed in minims, it is best to measure it in minims. The minim is measured with a minim glass; the drop, with a medicine dropper.

Numerical Symbols Commonly Used with the Apothecary System

ss̄ = ½
ī = 1
īī = 2
īīī = 3
īv̄ = 4
v̄ = 5

v̄ī = 6
v̄īī = 7
v̄īīī = 8
īx̄ = 9
x̄ = 10
x̄v̄ = 15

When apothecary symbols are used, the quantity is expressed in lower case Roman numerals, which are placed after the symbol: gr ii, ʒii, ʒiii. However, when fractions are indicated, or when

pt, qt, and gal are written Arabic numerals are always used: gr ¼, qt 9. The only exception to this rule is the quantity ½, which is expressed as the symbol ss̄ (Latin *semi* or *semisis,* meaning half).

MEDICATION AND I.V. BASICS

Approximate Metric and Apothecary Weight Equivalents

METRIC	APOTHECARY	METRIC	APOTHECARY
1 gram (g) (1,000 mg)	= 15 grains	0.05 g (50 mg)	= ¾ grain
		0.03 g (30 mg)	= ½ grain
0.6 g (600 mg)	= 10 grains	0.015 g (15 mg)	= ¼ grain
0.5 g (500 mg)	= 7½ grains	0.001 g (1 mg)	= ⅟₆₀ grain
0.3 g (300 mg)	= 5 grains	0.6 mg	= ⅟₁₀₀ grain
0.2 g (200 mg)	= 3 grains	0.5 mg	= ⅟₁₂₀ grain
0.1 g (100 mg)	= 1½ grains	0.4 mg	= ⅟₁₅₀ grain
0.06 g (60 mg)	= 1 grain		

Approximate Household, Apothecary, and Metric Volume Equivalents

HOUSEHOLD	APOTHECARY	METRIC
1 teaspoonful (tsp)	= 1 fluidram	= 4 or 5 ml*
1 tablespoonful (T or tbs)	= ½ fluidounce	= 15 ml
2 tablespoonfuls	= 1 fluidounce	= 30 ml
1 measuring cupful	= 8 fluidounces	= 240 ml
1 pint (pt)	= 16 fluidounces	= 473 ml
1 quart (qt)	= 32 fluidounces	= 946 ml
1 gallon (gal)	= 128 fluidounces	= 3,785 ml

*Although the fluidram is approximately 4 ml, in prescriptions it is considered equivalent to the teaspoon (which is 5 ml).

Calculations: Setting Up Proportions

Setting up a proportion may be the least complex method for converting measures either within the same system or from one system to another. A proportion is made up of two ratios, each indicating the relationship one quantity has to the other. It can be written as whole units or as a fraction:

$$A:B::C:D \text{ or } 2:3::4:6$$
$$\frac{A}{B}=\frac{C}{D} \text{ or } \frac{2}{3}=\frac{4}{6}$$

The first and fourth terms (A and D) are called the extremes, and the second and third terms (B and C) are called the means. The product of the means equals the product of the extremes.

$$2:3::4:6 \qquad \frac{2}{3}=\frac{4}{6}$$
$$2\times 6=3\times 4 \qquad 2\times 6=3\times 4$$
$$12=12 \qquad 12=12$$

The proportion method can be helpful when one of your terms is unknown (x).

• Keep the unknown quantity on the left, the known on the right.
• Solve the proportion by equating the product of the means to the product of the extremes.
• For the value of x, simply divide the numerical value of the product containing the x into the product on the right of the equation.

Example:
How many ampicillin capsules containing 250 mg each do you need to give 1 g?

Step 1: Convert the amount desired and the size of the tablet on hand into a common unit.
$$1 g = 1,000 \text{ mg}$$

Step 2: Set up a proportion.
$$\frac{mg}{caps}=\frac{mg}{caps}$$

Unknown   *Known*
$$\frac{1,000 \text{ mg}}{x \text{ capsules}} = \frac{250 \text{ mg}}{1 \text{ capsule}}$$

$$250\,x = 1,000$$

$$x = 4 \text{ capsules}$$

I.V. Fluid Calculations

When administering I.V. fluids, you must calculate and regulate the number of drops per minute to administer a prescribed amount of solution in a designated period of time. Maintaining proper flow rates for prescribed solutions is essential to prevent complications.

I.V. administration sets are constructed to deliver a specific number of drops per milliliter. This is called the drop factor and can be found on the package containing the set:

10 drops/ml—Baxter (Travenol)
13 drops/ml—McGaw
15 drops/ml—Abbott
20 drops/ml—Cutter; IVAC
60 drops/ml—microdrip

Example:
The doctor ordered 1,000 ml of dextrose 5% in water to be infused in 8 hours. What is the rate of infusion?

Step 1: Convert hours into minutes, since you will need to figure drops/minute.

Step 2: Set up a proportion using the available information.

$$\frac{minute}{ml} = \frac{minute}{ml}$$

Unknown   *Known*

$$\frac{1 \text{ minute}}{x \text{ ml}} = \frac{480 \text{ minutes}}{1,000 \text{ ml}}$$

$$480x = 1,000$$

$$x = 2.1 \text{ ml/minute}$$

Next, calculate the number of drops/minute:
● Note the number of drops/ml the I.V. set you have delivers (10, 13, 15, 20, or 60).
● Convert the number of milliliters to drops by multiplying the two figures.

Continued

I.V. Fluid Calculations
Continued

Examples:
Baxter set—10 drops/ml
2.1 ml/minute × 10 drops/
ml = 21 drops/minute

Abbott set—15 drops/ml
2.1 ml/minute × 15 drops/
ml = 32 drops/minute

*Short formula for determining
rate of infusion*

volume of solution
time interval in minutes
× drop factor = drops/minute

$\frac{1,000}{480}$(= 2.1 ml/minute)
× 15 (Abbott) = 32

Sometimes the doctor speci-
fies the volume of I.V. solution to
be infused each hour. In this
case, use the hourly volume,
not the container volume.

Example:
*The orders read, "Give 500 ml
dextrose 5% in water at 50 ml/
hour." The drop factor of your
I.V. microdrip set is 60 drops/ml.*

volume of solution
time interval in minutes
× drop factor = drops/minute

$\frac{50}{60}$× 60 = 50 drops/minute

Common Abbreviations

The following list shows some abbreviations you'll frequently encounter when administering medications.

a.c.	before eating	os	mouth, bone
b.i.d.	twice daily	oz	ounce
$\bar{c}$	with	paren.	parenterally
cc	cubic centimeter	p.c.	after meals
cm	centimeter	per	through, by
/d	daily	p.o.	by mouth
et	and	p.r.n.	as needed
Gm, gm	gram	pt	pint
gr	grain	p.v.	through the vagina
Gtt, gtt	drop	Q.h.	every hour
H	hour	Q.2h.	every 2 hours
h.n.	tonight	q.i.d.	four times a day
h.s.	at bedtime	q.s.	a sufficient quantity
hypo	hypodermically	qt	quart
I.M.	intramuscular, intramuscularly	$\bar{s}$	without
		s.c., s.cut.	subcutaneous, subcutaneously
IU	international unit		
I.V.	intravenous, intravenously	Sig.	write; label
kg	kilogram	$\overline{ss}$	half
L	liter	stat	immediately
m	meter, minim	t.i.d.	three times a day
mEq	milliequivalent	tinct.	tincture
mg	milligram	top.	topically
ml	milliliter	ung.	ointment
mm	millimeter		
O.D.	right eye		
O.L., O.S.	left eye		

Administering I.V. Therapy

I.V. therapy may be used for the administration of fluids (such as crystalloids, colloids, blood, and nutrients) and medications. Most fluids are infused continuously but, in some cases, may be infused intermittently. Medications can be introduced intravenously by continuous infusion; bolus infusion; or intermittent infusion, using methods such as the piggyback (secondary line) or intermittent infusion injection.

Follow these guidelines when administering I.V. therapy:
• Before administering any medication intravenously, consider possible incompatibility with fluids and other drugs given at the same time.
• Always clean the injection port with an alcohol swab or sponge before injecting medication, whether it's through a Y port of I.V. tubing, into an intermittent infusion device, or directly into an I.V. solution bottle or bag.
• Whenever giving I.V. injections of any type, always inspect the injection site for signs of extravasation and phlebitis.
• Change I.V. tubing and dressings according to hospital requirements, and apply antimicrobial ointment to the injection site. Record on the I.V. dressing and on the patient's chart the catheter (needle) type and gauge, date and time the catheter or needle was inserted, and your initials.
• Adverse reactions to substances administered I.V. can occur almost immediately. In such cases, discontinue administration immediately, and notify the doctor. Wherever I.V. therapy is used, emergency equipment and drugs should be readily available.
• Substances injected intravenously are absorbed into the system immediately. Take special care to prevent (or recognize) toxic reactions or shock caused by allergic reactions or by introducing too much solution too quickly.

The patient's condition and age, type of fluid or drug being administered, size of the administration set, and viscosity of the liquid itself are the principal factors determining the flow rate.

For greater accuracy, the flow rate should be measured in microdrops (requiring a special solution set) or regulated with an infusion control device.

Continued

Administering I.V. Therapy
Continued

The infusion should be administered in strict accordance with the doctor's instructions.

• Should the flow stop, first check for signs of infiltration. Then try to determine if the tubing is defective. Also, hold the bottle below the injection site level to backwash anything obstructing the flow.

If hospital procedure permits, irrigate catheter with 1 ml of sterile saline solution. Keep in mind that any filter being used may be clogged and may need to be changed.

• Administer supplemental drugs one at a time to prevent incompatibilities. Always flush the injection site on the tubing or intermittent infusion device with several milliliters of sterile saline solution between injections.

• If an intermittent infusion device is used for administration of a drug other than heparin, a small amount of dilute heparin solution is placed into the lock after drug injection and flushing to maintain patency. Always remember to flush this out of the lock before injecting another drug, as the two solutions may be incompatible.

• Many hospitals keep lists of drugs that may or may not be administered I.V. by nurses. If you work in such a hospital, become familiar with this list, and check with the pharmacist about any drugs you aren't familiar with.

• When not already prepackaged from the manufacturer, unit doses are best prepared, diluted, and labeled under sterile conditions by the pharmacist.

• If unit dose–packaged syringes aren't available, dilute the medication according to directions, using only the exact diluent recommended by the manufacturer. If you're working with sterile water for injection, remember that ampules are meant for single use only. Diluent in vials previously used for reconstitution of other drugs may be contaminated, so always use a fresh vial.

Many drugs prove irritating to the vein wall, but proper dilution can at least minimize such irritations.

Calculating Flow Rates

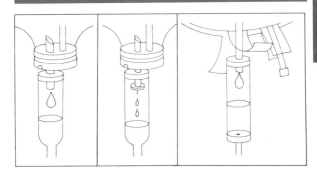

When calculating the flow rate of I.V. solutions, remember that the number of drops required to deliver 1 ml varies with the type of administration set used and the manufacturer. The illustration at top left shows a standard (macrodrip) set, which delivers from 10 to 20 drops/ml. The illustration in the top center shows a pediatric (microdrip) set, which delivers about 60 drops/ml. The illustration at top right shows a blood transfusion set, which delivers about 10 drops/ml.

To calculate the flow rate, it is necessary to know the calibration of the drip rate for each manufacturer's product. As a quick guide, refer to the chart on page 22. Use this formula to calculate specific drip rates.

$$\frac{\text{Volume of infusion (in ml)}}{\text{time of infusion (in minutes)}} \times \text{drop factor in drops/ml} = \text{drops/min}$$

Continued

MEDICATION AND I.V. BASICS

Calculating Flow Rates
Continued

CO. NAME	DROPS/ML	DROPS/MINUTE TO INFUSE					
		500 ml/ 24 hr	1,000 ml/ 24 hr	1,000 ml/ 20 hr	1,000 ml/ 10 hr	1,000 ml/ 8 hr	1,000 ml/ 6 hr
		21 ml/hr	42 ml/hr	50 ml/hr	100 ml/hr	125 ml/hr	166 ml/hr
Abbott-Baxter	15	5gtts	10 gtts	12 gtts	25 gtts	31 gtts	42 gtts
Travenol	10	3 gtts	7 gtts	8 gtts	17 gtts	21 gtts	28 gtts
Cutter	20	7 gtts	14 gtts	17 gtts	34 gtts	42 gtts	56 gtts
IVAC	20	7 gtts	14 gtts	17 gtts	34 gtts	42 gtts	56 gtts
McGaw	13	4 gtts	9 gtts	11 gtts	22 gtts	27 gtts	36 gtts
Microdrip	60	21 gtts	42 gtts	50 gtts	100 gtts	125 gtts	166 gtts

Giving Tablets and Capsules

Before you administer any medication, double-check the medication label with the doctor's order. Then, confirm the patient's identity by checking the wristband and asking the patient his name. Finally, wash your hands thoroughly, and remember to maintain clean technique throughout the procedure. Now, you're ready to begin.

• First, gather the equipment. If you plan to crush an uncoated tablet, you'll need a mortar and pestle or a commercially made pulverizer; if you plan to divide a scored tablet, you'll need a knife. But most of the time, all you'll need is the bottle of medication, a small soufflé cup or medicine cup, and water or juice.

• Pour the correct number of tablets or capsules into the bottle cap. If you pour out too many, put the excess back. *Important:* Never touch any excess medication, or you may contaminate the entire bottle. For the same reason, don't return the unused portion of a divided tablet to the bottle. Instead, discard it.

• Now, pour the tablets or capsules into the soufflé cup or medicine cup, and recap the medication bottle. Then, give the cup to the patient or tap the medication into his hand. Keep the water or juice nearby.

• Now, tell the patient to put the tablets or capsules well back on his tongue. (He may take them one at a time or all at once, whichever way he prefers.) If he can't do this himself, help him.

Important: Avoid touching the patient's mouth, or the rim of the medicine cup after he's used it. If you do, wash your hands immediately, so you don't transfer any bacteria to your next patient.

• Then, ask him to tip his head slightly forward and swallow a full mouthful of water or juice. Warn him not to throw his head back as he swallows. This position may prevent his airway from closing and may increase the risk of aspiration.

Finally, discard the used soufflé cup and document the procedure.

ORAL AND DERMATOMUCOSAL MEDICATIONS

What You Should Know About Crushing Tablets

If your patient has difficulty swallowing his medication, you may want to crush a tablet or open a capsule to make administration easier. But, to make sure you can *safely* do so, read the following guidelines.

Generally, you may crush tablets and open capsules. (Some capsules—for example, those containing pediatric doses—are specially designed to be opened.) Then you can mix the medication with a beverage or a small amount of soft food, such as applesauce or mashed potatoes, before administering it. But before mixing any medication with a food or beverage, be sure to check that the drug's action won't be affected. And since the medication may alter the food's taste, tell your patient what you've done.

But never crush a sustained-release or enteric-coated tablet. Remember,

the special coating is designed to ensure proper absorption at the right time, in the right place. If you crush a sustained-release tablet, the entire dose is available for absorption all at once, instead of over a period of hours. A drug overdose could result. Similarly, crushing an enteric-coated tablet destroys the drug's protective coating. As a result, the drug will dissolve in the stomach instead of the small intestine, possibly causing gastric irritation or even vomiting.

You may open a sustained-release *capsule* and mix its contents with food or water. But take care to mix the drug *gently,* not vigorously.

Note: Check with the pharmacist before crushing any tablets. He may be able to provide a liquid form of the drug or prepare a special formulation.

Understanding Liquid Oral Medications

SYRUP

Description
• A drug and preservative in a viscous, sugar/water solution; usually flavored

Special considerations
• When giving a syrup for a demulcent (soothing) effect, don't follow it with water. Tell the patient to sip the syrup slowly.
• When giving a syrup for a systemic effect, you may dilute it. However, dilute only the dose being given. If you dilute the entire bottle, you may destroy the preservative and hasten contamination or decomposition.
• Use caution when administering syrups to diabetic patients. Check with the pharmacist to see if a sugar-free syrup is available.
• When giving syrups with other drugs, be sure to administer syrups *last.*
• Remember, take special care to keep syrups out of the reach of children.

SUSPENSION

Description
• *Magma:* a thick, milky suspension of an insoluble (or partly soluble) inorganic drug, suspended in water
• *Gel:* the same as magma but with smaller drug particles
• *Emulsion:* droplets of fat or oil, suspended in water

Special considerations
• Always shake a suspension thoroughly before giving it.
• If desired, you may dilute most suspensions with water before administration. However, don't dilute an *antacid* suspension, or it won't coat the stomach effectively.

ALCOHOLIC SOLUTION

Description
• *Elixir:* a clear mixture of a drug, alcohol, water, and sugar; sweet-tasting. However, elixirs are not as sweet as syrups. They are also less viscous than syrups. Alcohol concentration ranges from 8% to 78%.

Continued

ORAL AND DERMATOMUCOSAL MEDICATIONS

Understanding Liquid Oral Medications
Continued

ALCOHOLIC SOLUTION
Continued

• *Spirits:* a solution of volatile substances; for example, liquids, solids, or gases. The alcohol in the solution acts as a preservative and solvent. The solution is used primarily as a flavoring agent.
• *Tincture:* a solution of alcohol, or alcohol and water, with animal or vegetable products or chemical substances.

Special considerations
• Check the solution carefully. Never administer one that has precipitate at the bottom of the bottle.
• If you want to dilute the solution, use only a small amount of water. More water could cause the drug to precipitate.
• Consult the pharmacist before you mix alcoholic solutions with liquids other than water.
• Follow administration with water, unless the solution's given for cough relief.

• Store solution in an airtight container. Protect from temperature extremes.
• Use these solutions cautiously if your patient is an alcoholic. *Important:* Never give an alcoholic solution to a patient receiving Antabuse.

RECONSTITUTED POWDERS AND TABLETS

Description
• Solid drugs reconstituted with water (or another suitable liquid) and given to the patient in suspension or solution form
Special considerations
• Read the directions carefully before reconstituting powders and tablets. Don't use too much water with effervescent tablets, or they'll boil out of the glass.
• Some powders will become gelatinous very quickly after you mix them. Administer them immediately after reconstitution.
• Wait until effervescent tablets dissolve completely before you give them to the patient. Give without further dilution.

Measuring Liquid Medication in a Disposable Medicine Cup

To begin, you'll need the bottle of medication, a disposable medicine cup and a damp paper towel. If you plan to dilute the medication, also obtain some water or juice. (However, make sure the medication's compatible with the diluent.)

Choose a disposable medicine cup that has all the markings you need. Never try to estimate measurements *between* markings, or your dosage won't be accurate. Check the bottle label against the Kardex.

• If the medication's a suspension, shake it well. Then, uncap the bottle, and place the cap upside down on a clean surface.

Rinse the medication cup in water. This will prevent medication from sticking to its sides.

• Locate the correct marking on the medicine cup. Keeping your thumbnail on the mark, hold the cup at eye level, and pour in the correct amount of medication. As you pour,

keep the label pointed up, so spilled liquid won't obscure it. Recheck the label against the Kardex.

• Now, recheck the dosage you've poured into the cup. To do this, set the cup on a level surface, and read the base of the meniscus at eye level. If you've poured too much medication into the cup, discard the excess. Don't return it to the bottle.

• Wipe the bottle lip with a damp paper towel, taking care not to touch the inside of the bottle. Replace the cap. Recheck the label against the Kardex.

• Now you're ready to give the medication to the patient. Position him comfortably in either a sitting or high Fowler's position. Hand him the cup of medication, and wait until he drinks it all.

• Discard the medicine cup, taking care not to touch the rim and contaminate your fingers. Finally, document the entire procedure.

Giving Medication with a Medication Syringe

ORAL AND DERMATOMUCOSAL
MEDICATIONS

• First, choose the proper syringe. Syringes vary in size. Some are marked in teaspoons as well as cubic centimeters or milliliters, and most are disposable. When choosing a syringe, consider the size of the dose, and the size and age of the patient. Always select a syringe that's marked precisely for your needs. Never try to estimate between markings.

• To avoid contaminating the medication bottle with the syringe, pour the medication into a medicine cup. Then, withdraw the prescribed amount from the cup, with the syringe. Discard the cup and any excess medication. Never return medication to the bottle. Or try this alternative: Put a sterile needle on the syringe, and withdraw the prescribed amount directly from the bottle. Then, discard the needle.

• Now, check the dosage. Hold the syringe at eye level, and read the measurement from the top edge of the rubber stopper. If you've withdrawn too much, squirt the excess into a sink or wastebasket. Don't return it to the bottle.

• Get ready to give the medication to your patient. Seat him upright or place him in a high Fowler's position. To minimize aspiration risk, place the syringe tip in the pocket between his cheek mucosa and his second molar. Instill the medication slowly. Then, discard the syringe, and document the procedure.

• If you're using a large-volume (50 ml or more) syringe, place a 2″ (5 cm) length of latex tubing on the syringe tip. Then, you can easily instill medication into the cheek pocket without putting the entire syringe into the patient's mouth. You'll find that this improvised syringe tip is especially handy for elderly, confused, or severely debilitated patients.

Food Effects on Drugs

Food in the stomach may speed up, retard, or sometimes even prevent drug absorption. And some foods may affect one drug one way and another a different way.

Drugs given orally go through several processes before entering systemic circulation. Tablets, for example, must disintegrate and dissolve before they can be absorbed through the intestinal mucosa. But tablet breakdown is affected by the stomach's pH, so when food changes the pH, the rate and degree of breakdown—and of drug absorption—may also change.

Food stimulates various body secretions, including gastric acid and bile. For this reason, acid-labile drugs should be taken on an empty stomach, when gastric acid secretions are minimal. Fat-soluble drugs, however, should be administered with meals because bile helps dissolve them.

Food delays stomach emptying, so a drug given with meals may remain in the stomach longer and have a delayed therapeutic effect. So if a rapid effect is important, you'll do better to administer the drug when the patient's stomach is empty.

But sometimes a food buffer may be useful. It can, for example, reduce the gastrointestinal distress, nausea, and mucosal damage caused by ulcerogenic drugs such as aspirin and indomethacin (Indocin).

Before you administer medications, check possible drug and food interactions. You may help patients reduce unpleasant drug side effects, such as nausea, vomiting, dyspepsia, and diarrhea. You may even improve patient compliance and reduce the length (and cost) of a patient's hospital stay.

ORAL AND DERMATOMUCOSAL
MEDICATIONS

Giving Medication by the Sublingual or Buccal Routes

Sublingual and buccal routes of administration are used when a rapid action is desired, or when a drug is specifically designed to be easily absorbed into blood vessels under the tongue (sublingual route) or between the cheek and gums (buccal route). Sublingual and buccal administration of certain drugs prevents their destruction or transformation in the stomach or small intestine. Examples are nitroglycerin, isosorbide dinitrate, and some male hormones. These medications take effect very quickly because the oral mucosa's thin epithelium and abundant vasculature allow direct absorption into the bloodstream.

For sublingual administration:
• Place the tablet under the patient's tongue.
• Instruct the patient to keep the medication in place until it dissolves completely to ensure absorption.
• Caution the patient against chewing the tablet or touching it with his tongue to prevent accidental swallowing.
• Tell the patient not to smoke before the medication has dissolved because nicotine's vasoconstrictive effects slow absorption.

For buccal administration:
• Place the tablet in the upper or lower buccal pouch, between the cheek and gum.
• Instruct the patient to close his mouth and hold the tablet there until it's absorbed.

Special considerations
• Tell the patient not to drink water or swallow excessively until the tablet is completely absorbed.
• Some buccal medications may cause mucosal irritation. Alternate sides of the mouth for repeat doses to prevent continuous irritation of the same site.

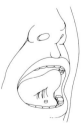

Sublingual route

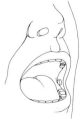

Buccal route

Giving Medication Through a Tube: General Guidelines

Whenever you give your patient medication through a gastric or a nasogastric tube, follow the same general procedure you learned for measuring and giving oral medications. For example, always double-check the order and observe the Five Rights. Also, don't neglect all the special considerations for the medication you're giving; for example, whether or not to give it with meals. Remember, the action of an oral medication doesn't change just because you're using a gastric or nasogastric tube.

Also, remember these guidelines:
• Give medication in liquid form only. If the prescribed medication is a tablet or capsule (and can be crushed or opened), mix it with juice, water, or another compatible liquid. Remember, the drug particles must be small enough to pass easily through the eyes of the tube.

Thoroughly mix the medication and liquid *before* pouring them into the syringe.
• Dilute any viscous liquid medication with water or another liquid, unless contraindicated or incompatible, *before* putting them in the syringe.
• Avoid giving an oily medication. It will cling to the sides of the tube and resist mixing with the flush solution.
• If you're giving the medication with a meal, give all the medication first—if the patient can't tolerate an entire feeding, you may have to stop the procedure before he receives the medication.
• Never give an adult more than 400 ml of liquid at a time. Never give an infant more than 120 ml of liquid at a time.
• Record the date and time of instillation, the dose, and the patient's tolerance of the procedure on the patient's record. Note the amount of fluid instilled on his intake and output sheet.

Administering Medication Through a Nasogastric Tube

ORAL AND DERMATOMUCOSAL
MEDICATIONS

Besides providing an alternate means of nourishment, the nasogastric (NG) tube allows direct instillation of medication into the GI system of patients who can't ingest it orally. Before instillation, the tube's patency and positioning must be carefully checked, since this procedure's contraindicated if the tube's obstructed or improperly positioned or if the patient is vomiting around the tube or has absent bowel sounds.

Oily medications and enteric-coated or sustained-release tablets shouldn't be instilled through an NG tube. Oily medications cling to the sides of the tube and resist mixing with the irrigating solution. Crushing enteric-coated or sustained-release tablets destroys their intended effect.

Follow these guidelines when administering medication through an NG tube:
• If necessary, prepare the medication.
• If the prescribed medication is in tablet form, crush the tablets to ready them for mixing with the diluting liquid. Make sure the particles are small enough to pass through the eyes at the tube's distal end.
• Explain the procedure to the patient, if necessary, and provide privacy.

• Confirm the patient's identity by asking his name and checking the name, room number, and bed number on his wristband.
• Unpin the tube from the patient's gown, and remove any dressing at the tube's end. To avoid soiling the sheets during the procedure, fold back the bed linens to the patient's waist and drape his chest with the towel or linen-saver pad.
• Elevate the head of the bed so the patient's in Fowler's or semi-Fowler's position.
• After removing the clamp from the tube, take a bulb or piston syringe and create a 10-cc air space in its chamber. Then attach the syringe to the tube's end.
• Auscultate the patient's abdomen about 3″ (8 cm) below the sternum with the stethoscope. Then, gently insert the 10 cc of air into the tube. You should hear the air bubble entering the stomach. If you hear this sound, gently draw back on the syringe. The appearance of gastric contents confirms that the tube's patent and in the stomach.
• If you meet resistance when aspirating for stomach contents, stop the procedure. Resistance may indicate a nonpatent tube or improper tube placement. To re-

Continued

Administering Medication Through a Nasogastric Tube
Continued

lieve resistance, withdraw the tube slightly.

• After you have established tube patency and correct positioning, hold the tube at a level slightly above the patient's nose and pour 30 ml of the diluted medication into the syringe barrel. To prevent air from entering the patient's stomach, hold the tube at a slight angle. If necessary, raise the tube slightly higher to increase the flow rate.

• If the medication flows smoothly, slowly add more until the entire dose has been given. To prevent air from entering the patient's stomach, add more medication before the syringe empties completely.

• If the medication doesn't flow properly, don't force it. It may be too thick to flow through the tube. If so, dilute it with water. If you suspect tube placement's inhibiting flow, stop the procedure and reevaluate the placement.

• Watch the patient's reaction throughout the instillation. If he shows any sign of discomfort, stop the procedure immediately.

• As the last of the medication flows out of the syringe, start to irrigate the tube by adding 50 ml of water. Irrigation clears medication from the tube's sides and dis-

tal end, reducing the risk of clogging.

• When the water stops flowing, quickly clamp the tube. Detach the syringe from the tube and dispose of it properly.

• Cover the end of the tube with a 4″ × 4″ sponge and secure it with the rubber band. Repin the tube to the patient's gown.

• Leave the patient in Fowler's or semi-Fowler's position for at least 30 minutes after the procedure to facilitate the downward flow of medication into his stomach and prevent reflux into the esophagus.

Special considerations

• To prevent instillation of too much fluid (more than 400 ml of liquid at one time for an adult), plan the drug instillation, if possible, so it doesn't coincide with the patient's regular tube feeding. When you must schedule both simultaneously, give the medication first to ensure that the patient receives prescribed drug therapy even if he can't tolerate an entire feeding.

• Liquids should be at room temperature. Administering cold liquid through the NG tube can cause abdominal cramping.

Administering Medication Through a Gastrostomy Tube

ORAL AND DERMATOMUCOSAL
MEDICATIONS

A gastrostomy tube provides a means for administering nutrients and medications to patients who can't ingest them orally. A gastrostomy tube, surgically inserted directly into the stomach, eliminates the risk of fluid aspiration into the lungs, a constant danger with a nasogastric tube. It also allows long-term use—the general indication for this procedure. Before instilling medication through a gastrostomy tube, check tube patency; warm or cool fluids to room temperature.

Note: This procedure's contraindicated in patients with absent bowel sounds or an obstructed tube. Follow these guidelines when administering medication through a gastrostomy tube:

• Crush the tablet or open the capsule to prepare the medication for mixing with the diluting liquid. Mix the medication with the appropriate amount of diluting liquid (usually 30 ml) and stir with the spoon.

• Confirm the patient's identity by asking his name and checking the name, room number, and bed number on his wristband.

• After closing the door or drawing the curtain to ensure privacy, explain the procedure to the patient.

• To avoid soiling the sheets during the procedure, fold the bed linens below the gastrostomy tube and drape the patient's chest with the towel or linen-saver pad.

• To facilitate digestion and prevent fluid reflux into the esophagus, elevate the head of the bed before instilling any medication.

• Remove the dressing that covers the tube. Then remove the dressing at the tip of the tube and attach the syringe or funnel to the tip.

Continued

Administering Medication Through a Gastrostomy Tube
Continued

• Release the clamp and instill about 10 ml of water into the tube through the syringe to check for patency. If the water flows in easily, the tube is patent. If it flows in slowly, raise the funnel to increase pressure. If the water still doesn't flow properly, stop the procedure and notify the doctor.

• Pour 30 ml of the medication at a time into the syringe or funnel. Tilt the tube to allow air to escape as the fluid flows downward.

• After the medication drains through the syringe or funnel, pour in about 30 ml of water to irrigate the tube.

• Tighten the clamp, then place one 4″ × 4″ gauze sponge on the end of the tube and secure it with a rubber band.

• Cover the tube with two 4″ × 4″ gauze sponges and secure it firmly with tape.

• Remove the towel or linen-saver pad and replace the bed linens.

• Keep the head of the bed elevated for at least 30 minutes after the procedure to aid digestion.

Special considerations
• Before pouring medication into the tube, gently lift the dressings around the tube to assess the skin for irritation caused by gastric secretions. Report any redness or irritation to the doctor.

• If the patient's stomach is already full, the liquid instilled can cause cramping and abdominal discomfort.

Guide to Rectal Medications

SUPPOSITORY

Description

A solid medication in a firm base, such as cocoa butter, that melts at body temperature. May be molded in a variety of cylindrical shapes. Usually about 1½″ (4 cm) long (smaller for infants and children).

Type for local use
- Analgesics
- Astringents
- Antipruritics
- Anti-inflammatories
- Laxatives, lubricants, and cathartics
- Carminatives

Type for systemic use
- Analgesics
- Antiemetics
- Antipyretics
- Bronchodilators
- Sedatives
- Hypnotics

OINTMENT

Description

A semisolid medication that may be applied externally to the anus or internally to the rectum.

Type for local use
- Antipruritics
- Astringents
- Analgesics and anesthetics
- Anti-inflammatories
- Antiseptics

Type for systemic use
- None

ENEMA

Description

Liquid given as either a *retention* enema (retained by the patient for at least 30 minutes or until absorbed) or a *nonretention* enema (retained by the patient for at least 10 minutes and then expelled). *Note:* Enemas given to cleanse the lower bowel aren't usually medicated.

Type for local use
- Anthelmintics
- Astringents
- Laxatives, lubricants, and cathartics
- Antiseptics
- Steroids

Type for systemic use
- Antipyretics
- Sedatives
- Anesthetics
- Nutritives and water

Administering Rectal Suppositories

A rectal suppository is a small, solid, medicated mass—usually cone-shaped—with a cocoa butter or glycerin base. It may be inserted to stimulate peristalsis and defecation or to relieve pain, vomiting, and local irritation. Rectal suppositories commonly contain drugs that reduce fever, induce relaxation, are impaired by digestive enzymes, or have a taste too offensive for oral use. Rectal suppositories melt at body temperature and are absorbed slowly.

Because insertion of a rectal suppository may stimulate the vagus nerve, this procedure's contraindicated in patients with potential cardiac dysrhythmias. It may have to be avoided in patients with recent rectal or prostate surgery because of the risk of local trauma or discomfort during insertion.

Follow these guidelines when administering a rectal suppository:
● Confirm the patient's identity by asking his name and checking the name, room number, and bed number on his wristband.
● Explain the procedure and the purpose of the medication to the patient.
● Provide privacy.
● Place the patient on his left side in the Sims' position. Drape him with the bedcovers to expose only the rectal area.
● Put a finger cot on the index finger of your dominant hand. (If a finger cot isn't readily available, use a glove.)
● Remove the suppository from its wrapper, and lubricate it with water-soluble lubricant.
● Lift the patient's upper buttock with your nondominant hand to expose the anus.
● Instruct the patient to take several deep breaths through his mouth to help relax the anal sphincters and reduce anxiety or discomfort during insertion.
● Using the index finger of your dominant hand, insert the suppository—tapered end first—about 1″ to 1½″ (2.5 to 4 cm), until you feel it pass the internal anal sphincter. Try to direct the tapered end toward the side of the rectum, so it contacts the membranes.
● Ensure the patient's comfort. Encourage him to lie quietly and, if applicable, to retain the suppository for the appropriate time period.

Special considerations
● Keep rectal suppositories stored in the refrigerator until needed to prevent softening and possible decreased effectiveness of medication. A softened suppository's also difficult to handle and insert. To harden it again, hold the suppository (in its wrapper) under cold running water. Advise the patient that the suppository may discolor his next bowel movement.

Guide to Enemas

Use this chart as a guide when you give your patient an enema. But before you decide which guidelines are appropriate, consider the type of medication the doctor has prescribed, as well as your patient's age, size, and condition. For instance, if your patient's a small 9-year-old, use the smallest tube suggested for his age-group. Physical size is more important than age.

Always use smaller tubing and less solution when you give a retention enema. This combination will create less pressure in the patient's rectum and make retention easier. *Note:* Never give a retention enema to an infant or young child. Neither will be able to retain it.

RETENTION ENEMAS

AGE-GROUP	RECTAL TUBE SIZE	TUBE AMOUNT TO INSERT	FLUID AMOUNT TO INTRODUCE
Adults	#14 to #20 French	3″ to 4″ (8 to 10 cm)	150 to 200 ml
Children over age 6	#12 to #14 French	2″ to 3″ (5 to 8 cm)	75 to 150 ml

NONRETENTION ENEMAS

AGE-GROUP	RECTAL TUBE SIZE	TUBE AMOUNT TO INSERT	FLUID AMOUNT TO INTRODUCE
Adults	#22 to #30 French	3″ to 4″ (8 to 10 cm)	750 to 1,000 ml
Children over age 6	#14 to #18 French	2″ to 3″ (5 to 8 cm)	500 to 1,000 ml
Children over age 2	#12 to #14 French	1½″ to 2″ (4 to 5 cm)	500 ml or less
Infants	#12 French	1″ to 1½″ (2.5 to 4 cm)	250 ml or less

Giving a Medicated Retention Enema

Medicated retention enemas of oil, magnesium sulfate, or glycerin and water are used for constipation, flatulence, and impaction. Sodium polystyrene sulfonate (Kayexalate) enemas treat hyperkalemia; neomycin enemas reduce intestinal bacteria that produce nitrogenous substances harmful to patients in hepatic coma.

Always take enough time to thoroughly prepare your patient before giving him a medicated retention enema. Make sure he understands the purpose of the enema and the importance of retaining the medication until it's absorbed. Schedule the procedure before meals—a full stomach triggers peristalsis, making retention more difficult.

To reduce the risk of stimulating peristalsis during the procedure, ask the patient to empty his bladder and rectum before you begin.

Before giving the enema, check your patient's condition. Notify the doctor if:
• your patient's constipated. Feces in his rectum will interfere with drug absorption.
• your patient has diarrhea. In this case, the drug may be expelled before it can be absorbed.
• your patient has an inflamed rectum. An enema may exacerbate the condition.

When giving a Kayexalate enema, keep these additional points in mind:

• Mix polystyrene resin only with water and sorbitol. Ion exchange requires an aqueous medium, and sorbitol prevents impaction. Ideally, this mixture should be administered orally. However, it may also be administered as a retention enema.
• Prevent fecal impaction in the elderly by administering resin rectally rather than orally. Give a cleansing enema first. Explain to the patient the necessity of retaining the Kayexalate enema. Retention for 6 to 10 hours is ideal, but 30 to 60 minutes is acceptable.
• Make sure the mixture's at body temperature to ensure patient comfort and to avoid stimulating peristalsis. But don't heat resin, as this impairs the drug's effectiveness.
• With the patient in Sims' position, insert a #28 French rubber catheter or a rectal tube about 10 cm (4") into the patient's sigmoid colon. Tape the tube in place.
• Agitate resin emulsion gently during administration to prevent settling.
• After administration, flush the tubing with 50 ml of water to ensure full delivery of medication.
• If back leakage occurs, place the patient in knee-chest position or elevate his hips.
• To help the patient with poor sphincter control retain the enema, consider using (if hospital policy permits) a Foley catheter with a 30-ml balloon inflated distal to the anal sphincter.

Administering Vaginal Medications

Vaginal medications include suppositories, creams, gels, and ointments. These medications can be inserted as topical treatment for infection or inflammation, or as a contraceptive. Suppositories have a cocoa butter base, which allows them to melt when they contact the vaginal mucosa and then diffuse topically, as effectively as creams, gels, and ointments.

Vaginal medications usually come with a disposable applicator that allows medication placement in the anterior and posterior fornices. Vaginal administration is most effective when the patient can remain lying down afterward and retain the medication.

Follow these guidelines when administering vaginal medication:
• Confirm the patient's identity by asking her name and checking the name, room number, and bed number on her wristband.
• Ask the patient to void.
• Ask the patient if she would rather insert the medication herself. If so, provide appropriate instructions. If not, proceed with the following steps.

To insert a suppository:
• Remove the suppository from the wrapper, and lubricate it with water-soluble lubricant.
• Put on gloves and expose the vagina.
• With the forefinger of your free hand, insert the suppository

about 2″ (5 cm) into the vagina. To ensure patient comfort, direct your finger *down* initially (toward the spine), and then *up* and *back* (toward the cervix).
• If the suppository is small, insert it in the tip of an applicator. Then, lubricate the applicator, hold it by the cylinder, and insert it into the vagina. When the suppository reaches the distal end of the vagina, depress the plunger. Remove the applicator while the plunger is still depressed.

To insert ointments, creams, or gels:
• Insert the plunger into the applicator. Then, fit the applicator to the tube of medication.
• Gently squeeze the tube to fill the applicator with the prescribed amount of medication. Lubricate the applicator.
• Put on gloves and expose the vagina.
• Insert the applicator as you would a small suppository and administer the medication.

Special considerations
Refrigerate vaginal suppositories that melt at room temperature.
• To prevent the medication from soiling the patient's clothing and bedding, provide a sanitary pad.
• Instruct the patient not to wear a tampon after inserting vaginal medication, because it would absorb the medication and decrease its effectiveness.

Guide to Topical Dosage Forms

This chart will tell you how topical dosage forms differ and how these differences affect your nursing care.

POWDER

Description
An inert chemical that may contain medication

Use
• Promotes skin drying
• Reduces moisture, maceration, friction

Special considerations
• Apply to clean, dry skin.
• To prevent inhalation of powder particles, instruct patient to turn his head to one side during application.
• If you're applying powder to the patient's face or neck, give him a cloth or gauze to cover his mouth. Then, ask him to exhale as you apply powder.

LOTION

Description
A suspension of insoluble powder in water or an emulsion without powder

Use
• Creates sensation of dryness
• Leaves uniform surface film of powder

• Soothes, cools, protects the skin

Special considerations
• Shake container well before using.
• Remove residue from previous applications, if ordered.
• To increase absorption in certain skin conditions, warm the patient's skin with heat packs or a bath before applying.
• Apply medication to clean, dry skin.
• Thoroughly massage lotion into the skin.
• After application, observe the patient's skin for local irritation.

CREAM

Description
An oil-in-water emulsion in semi-solid form

Use
• Lubricates as a barrier

Special considerations
• Remove residue from previous applications, if ordered.
• Apply medication to clean, dry skin.
• Thoroughly massage cream into the skin.
• After application, observe the patient's skin for local irritation.

Continued

Guide to Topical Dosage Forms
Continued

OINTMENT

Description
A suspension of oil and water in semisolid form
Use
• Retains body heat
• Provides prolonged medication contact
Special considerations
• Remove residue from previous applications, if ordered.
• To increase absorption of medication, warm patient's skin with heat packs or a bath before applying.
• Apply medication to clean, dry skin.
• Apply thin layer of ointment to patient's skin, and rub it in well.

• Use care when applying ointment to draining wounds.

PASTE

Description
A stiff mixture of powder and ointment
Use
• Provides a uniform coat
• Reduces and repels moisture
Special considerations
• Remove residue from previous applications, if ordered.
• Apply medication to clean, dry skin.
• Cover medication to increase absorption and to protect the patient's clothing and bed linen.

Topical Medications: Pros and Cons

Benefits
• Faster relief from surface pain and itching than with systemic drugs
• Less severe allergic reactions than with systemic drugs
• Fewer side effects than with systemic drugs
• Comforting for the patient, since he can witness the care
• Increased protection against infection for skin that's lost its natural protection capabilities

Drawbacks
• Difficult to deliver in precise doses
• May stain skin, clothing, furniture, or bed linen
• Application procedure is time-consuming
• May be embarrassing to patient, depending on the site
• May be difficult for the patient to apply, depending on the site

Applying Nitroglycerin Ointment

Unlike other medications applied to the skin, nitroglycerin ointment causes a systemic vasodilation rather than a local effect. Continuously absorbed through the skin into the circulation, it's effective for about 4 hours.

Follow these guidelines when applying nitroglycerin ointment:

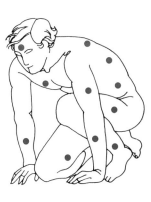

• Select an application site, such as the chest, arm, thigh, abdomen, forehead, ankle, or back. Choose a new site each time you apply a new dose to prevent minor skin irritations. Remove any traces of ointment left from previous applications.

• Using the ruled applicator paper that comes with the ointment, squeeze the prescribed ointment amount onto the paper.

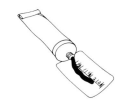

Continued

Applying Nitroglycerin Ointment
Continued

• Use the applicator paper to apply the ointment in a thin, uniform layer over an area of about 3″ to 6″ (8 to 15 cm). Leave the applicator paper on the site.

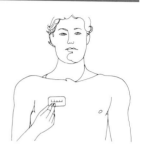

• Cover the applicator paper with plastic wrap and secure it with tape. This will protect clothing and ensure maximum absorption.

Special considerations
• If your patient experiences adverse effects, such as headache, dizziness, or faintness, notify the doctor—he may want to decrease the dose.
• To avoid coming into contact with nitroglycerin, which could lead to systemic absorption, you may want to wear gloves when applying the ointment.

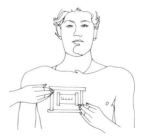

Applying Transdermal Medication

Through an adhesive disk or measured dose of ointment applied to the skin, transdermal medications supply constant, controlled medication directly into the bloodstream for prolonged systemic effect. The only medications currently available in transdermal form are nitroglycerin, used to control angina, and scopolamine, used to treat motion sickness. Most other medications have molecules too large for absorption through the skin. Nitroglycerin ointment dilates coronary vessels for up to 4 hours; a nitroglycerin disk can produce the same effect for as long as 24 hours. The scopolamine disk can relieve motion sickness for as long as 72 hours.

Contraindications for transdermal application include skin allergies or skin reactions to the medication. Transdermal medications should not be applied to broken or irritated skin because they would increase irritation, or to scarred or callused skin, which may impair absorption.

To apply transdermal ointments:
• Place the prescribed amount of ointment on the application strip or measuring paper, taking care not to get any on your skin.
• Apply the strip to any dry and, if possible, hairless body area. Don't rub the ointment into the skin.
• Tape the application strip and ointment to the skin.
• If desired, cover the application strip with the plastic wrap, and tape the wrap in place.

To apply transdermal disks:
• Open the package and remove the disk.
• Without touching the adhesive surface, remove the clear-plastic backing.
• Apply the disk to a dry, hairless area (scopolamine is usually applied behind the ear).

After applying transdermal medications:
• Instruct the patient to keep the area around the disk or ointment as dry as possible.
• Wash your hands immediately after applying the disk or ointment to avoid absorbing the medication yourself.

Special considerations
• Reapply daily transdermal medications at the same time every day to ensure a continuous effect, but alternate the application sites to avoid skin irritation. Before reapplying nitroglycerin ointment, remove the plastic wrap, application strip, and any remaining ointment from the patient's skin.
• When applying a scopolamine disk, instruct the patient not to drive or operate machinery until his response to the medication has been determined.
• Skin irritation, such as pruritus or a rash, may occur.

Applying a Nitroglycerin Disk

Nitroglycerin relieves anginal pain by temporarily dilating (widening) veins and arteries. This brings more blood and oxygen to the heart when it needs it most, reducing the heart's work load.

A nitroglycerin disk consists of a gel-like substance attached to an adhesive bandage. When applied to the skin, the disk allows nitroglycerin to be absorbed through the skin into the bloodstream. A single application lasts 24 hours.

Apply the disk to any convenient skin area—preferably on the upper arm or chest—without touching the gel or surrounding tape. Use a different site every day to avoid skin irritation. If necessary, you can shave an appropriate site. Avoid any area that may cause uneven absorption,

such as skin folds, scars, and calluses, or any irritated or damaged skin areas. Also, don't apply the disk below the elbow or knee.

After application, wash your hands to remove any nitroglycerin that may have rubbed off.

Tell the patient to try not to get the disk wet when he showers. If the disk should leak or fall off, throw it away. Then, clean the site and apply a new disk at a different site.

To ensure 24-hour coverage, apply the nitroglycerin disk at the same time every day. Bedtime application is ideal, because body movement is at a minimum during the night. Also, to ensure continuous nitroglycerin therapy, apply a new disk about 30 minutes before removing the old one.

Administering Eye Medications

Eye medications—drops, ointments, and disks—may be used diagnostically or therapeutically. During an eye examination, eye drops can be used to anesthetize the eye, dilate the pupil to facilitate retraction, and stain the cornea to identify corneal abrasions and scars. Eye medications may also be used to lubricate the eye and treat certain eye conditions.

Follow these guidelines when administering eye medications:

• Use sterile technique to avoid eye irritation or infection. All equipment and medication must also be sterile.

• Make sure the medication's labeled for ophthalmic use. Then check the expiration date. Remember to date the container the first time you use the medication. Usually, an eye medication may be used for a maximum of 2 weeks.

• Inspect eye solutions for cloudiness, discoloration, and precipitation, but remember that some eye medications normally appear cloudy. Don't use any solution that appears abnormal. If the tip of an eye ointment tube has crusted, turn the tip on a sterile gauze pad to remove the crust.

• Before instilling the medication, remove any discharge by cleansing around the eye with cotton balls moistened with warm water or normal saline solution. With the patient's eye closed, cleanse from the inner canthus to the outer canthus, using a fresh cotton ball for each stroke.

• To remove crusted secretions around the eye, moisten a gauze pad with warm water or normal saline solution. Ask the patient to close the eye, then place the gauze pad over it for a minute or two. Remove the pad, then reapply moist sterile gauze pads, as necessary, until the secretions are soft enough to be removed without traumatizing the mucosa.

• Have the patient sit or lie in the supine position. Instruct him to tilt his head back and toward the side of the affected eye so excess solution can flow away from the tear duct, preventing systemic absorption through the nasal mucosa.

• Remove the dropper cap from the medication container. Be careful to avoid contaminating the bottle top. Fill the dropper, as necessary.

• Before instilling the eye drops, instruct the patient to look up and away. This moves the cornea away from the lower lid and minimizes the risk of touching the cornea with the dropper if the patient blinks.

• Gently pull down the lower lid to expose the conjunctival sac.

Continued

ORAL AND DERMATOMUCOSAL MEDICATIONS

Administering Eye Medications
Continued

ORAL AND DERMATOMUCOSAL MEDICATIONS

To instill eye drops:

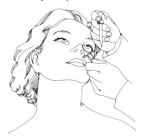

• Steady the hand in which you are holding the dropper against the patient's forehead. Then, with your other hand, gently pull down the lower lid of the affected eye and instill the drops in the conjunctival sac. Never instill eye drops directly onto the eyeball.
• Instruct the patient to close his eyes gently, without squeezing the lids shut. Then tell him to blink.
• Remove any excess solution surrounding the eye with a clean tissue. Use a separate tissue for each eye.
• Apply a new eye dressing, if necessary.

To apply eye ointment:
• Squeeze a small ribbon of medication on the conjunctival sac from the inner canthus to the outer canthus. Cut off the ribbon by turning the tube. If you wish, you can steady the hand holding the medication tube by bracing it against the patient's forehead or cheek.
• Instruct the patient to close his eyes gently, without squeezing the lids shut. Then tell him to roll his eyes to help distribute the ointment over the eyeball's surface.
• Remove any excess ointment surrounding the eyes with a clean tissue. Use a separate tissue for each eye.
• Apply a new dressing, if indicated.

Special considerations
When administering an eye medication that may be absorbed systemically (such as atropine), gently place your thumb over the inner canthus for 1 to 2 minutes after instilling drops, while the patient closes his eyes. This helps prevent medication from flowing into the tear duct.

Discard any solution remaining in the dropper before returning it to the bottle. If the dropper has become contaminated, discard it and obtain another sterile dropper. To avoid cross-infection, never use a container of eye medication for more than one patient.

Inserting and Removing an Eye Medication Disk

A medication disk inserted into the eye can release medication for up to 1 week. Pilocarpine, for example, can be administered this way to treat glaucoma. The small, flexible oval disk consists of three layers: two soft outer layers and a middle layer containing the medication. Floating between the eyelids and the sclera, the disk stays in the eye while the patient sleeps and even during swimming and athletic activities. Once the disk is in place, the fluid in the eye moistens it, releasing the medication. Eye moisture or contact lenses don't adversely affect the disk. Eye medication disks offer the advantage of continuous release of medication. Contraindications include conjunctivitis, keratitis, retinal detachment, and any condition where constriction of the pupil should be avoided.

To insert an eye medication disk:

● Arrange to insert the disk before the patient goes to bed. This minimizes the problems caused by blurring after the disk is inserted.

● Wash your hands.
● Press your fingertip against the oval disk so its length lies horizontally across your fingertip. It should stick to your finger. Lift it out of its packet.
● Evert the patient's lower eyelid, and place the disk in the conjunctival sac. It should lie horizontally, not vertically. The disk will automatically stick to the eye.
● Pull the lower eyelid out, up, and over the disk. Tell the patient to blink several times. If the disk is still visible, lift the lower lid out and over the disk again. Tell the patient that once the disk is in place, he can adjust its position by *gently* pressing his finger against his closed lid. Caution him against rubbing his eye or moving the disk across the iris.
● If the disk falls out, wash your hands, rinse the disk in cool water, and reinsert it. If the disk bends out of shape, replace it. If both of the patient's eyes are being treated with medication disks, replace both disks at the same time, so both eyes receive medication at the same rate.
Continued

Inserting and Removing an Eye Medication Disk
Continued

• If the disk continually slips out of position, reinsert the disk under the upper eyelid. To do this, gently lift and evert the upper eyelid and insert the disk in the conjunctival sac. Then, gently pull the lid back into position and tell the patient to blink several times. To adjust the disk to the most comfortable position, have the patient gently press on the closed lid. The more the patient uses the disk, the easier it should be for him to retain it. If he can't, notify the doctor.

• Before discharge, if the patient will continue therapy with an eye medication disk, teach him to insert and remove it himself. To check his mastery of these skills, have him insert and remove it for you.

• Also, teach the patient about possible side effects. Foreign-body sensation in the eye, mild tearing or redness, increased mucous discharge, eyelid redness, and itchiness can occur with the use of disks. Blurred vision, stinging, swelling, and headaches can occur with pilocarpine, specifically. Mild symptoms are common but should subside within the first 6 weeks of use. Tell the patient to report persistent or severe symptoms to his doctor.

To remove an eye medication disk:

• You can remove an eye medication disk with one or two fingers. To use *one finger,* evert the lower eyelid with one hand so you expose the disk. Then, use the forefinger of your other hand to slide the disk onto the lid and out of the patient's eye. To use *two fingers,* evert the lower lid with one hand to expose the disk. Then, pinch the disk with the thumb and forefinger of your other hand and remove it from the eye.

• If the disk is in the upper eyelid, apply long circular strokes to the patient's closed eyelid with your finger until you can see the disk in the corner of the patient's eye. Once the disk is visible, place your finger directly on the disk and move it to the lower sclera. Then remove it as you would a disk in the lower lid.

Instilling Ear Drops

Ear drops may be instilled to treat infection and inflammation, to soften cerumen for later removal, to produce local anesthetic effects, or to facilitate removal of an insect trapped in the ear by immobilizing and smothering it. Instillation of ear drops is usually contraindicated if the patient has a perforated eardrum; however, it may be permitted with certain medications, but then requires sterile technique. Other conditions may also prohibit instillation of certain other medications into the ear. For instance, instillation of drops containing hydrocortisone is contraindicated if the patient has herpes, another viral infection, or a fungal infection.

Follow these guidelines when administering ear drops:

• To avoid side effects (such as vertigo, nausea, and pain) resulting from instillation of excessively cold ear drops, warm the medication to body temperature in a bowl of warm water or carry it in your pocket for 30 minutes before administration. If necessary, test the medication's temperature by placing a drop on your wrist. (If it's too hot, it may burn the patient's eardrum or, at the very least, be ineffective.) Before using a glass dropper, make sure it's not chipped to avoid injury to the ear canal.

• Position the patient to lie on his side opposite the affected ear.

• Straighten the patient's ear canal. For an adult, pull the ear's auricle up and back. For an infant or a child under age 3, gently pull the auricle down and back (the ear canal's straighter at this age).

• Using a light source, examine the ear canal for drainage. If you find any drainage, clean it with a tissue or cotton-tipped applicator because drainage can interfere with the medication's effectiveness.

• To avoid damaging the ear canal with the dropper, gently

ORAL AND DERMATOMUCOSAL MEDICATIONS

Continued

Instilling Ear Drops
Continued

ORAL AND DERMATOMUCOSAL
MEDICATIONS

support the hand holding the dropper against the patient's head. Straighten the patient's ear canal once again and instill the number of drops ordered. To avoid patient discomfort, direct the drops to fall against the sides of the ear canal, not on the eardrum.

• Instruct the patient to remain on his side for 5 to 10 minutes to allow the medication to run down into the ear canal.

• If ordered, tuck a cotton ball loosely into the ear canal opening to prevent the medication from leaking out. Be careful not to insert it too deeply into the canal because this would prevent drainage of secretions and increase pressure on the eardrum.

• Clean and dry the outer ear.

Special considerations

Remember that some conditions make the normally tender ear canal even more sensitive, so be especially gentle when performing this procedure. Remember, to prevent injury to the eardrum, never insert a cotton-tipped applicator into the ear canal past the point where you can see the tip.

Remember to always wash your hands before and after caring for the patient's ear and between caring for both ears. Strict asepsis is especially vital if the patient's middle or inner ear has been opened by surgery or trauma.

Instilling Nasal Medications

Nasal medications may be instilled by means of drops, a spray (atomizer), or an aerosol (nebulizer). Most drugs instilled by these methods produce local rather than systemic effects. Drops can be directed at a specific area; sprays and aerosols diffuse medication throughout the nose.

To instill nose drops:
• When possible, position the patient so the drops flow back into the nostrils, toward the affected area. If you want the drops to reach the eustachian tube opening, place the patient in supine position, with his head tilted slightly to the affected side. To reach the ethmoidal and the sphenoidal sinuses, place the patient in the Proetz position (with his head hanging over the edge of the bed). To reach the maxillary and the frontal sinuses and the nasal passages, place the patient in the Parkinson position (with his head toward the affected side and hanging slightly over the edge of the bed).
• If the patient can't assume either the Proetz or the Parkinson position, position him supine, and put a large pillow under his shoulders so the head tilts back over the shoulders. Tilt the head as far back as possible to prevent the drops from running into the throat.

• Draw up some medication into the dropper.
• Push up the tip of the patient's nose slightly. Position the dropper just above the nostril, and direct its tip toward the midline of the nose, so the drops flow toward the back of the nasal cavity rather than toward its base, where they would flow down the throat.
• Insert the dropper about ⅜″ (1 cm) into the nostril. Make sure the dropper doesn't touch the sides of the nostril, because this would contaminate the dropper and could cause the patient to sneeze.

Nose drops

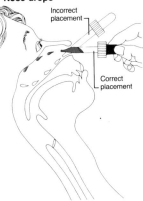

Incorrect placement

Correct placement

Continued

ORAL AND DERMATOMUCOSAL MEDICATIONS

Instilling Nasal Medications
Continued

• Instill the prescribed number of drops, observing the patient carefully for any signs of discomfort.
• To prevent the drops from leaking out of the nostrils, ask the patient to keep his head tilted back for at least 5 minutes and to breathe through his mouth. This also allows sufficient time for the medication to constrict mucous membranes.

To use a nasal spray:
• Have the patient sit upright, with his head tilted back slightly.
• Remove the protective cap from the atomizer.
• To prevent air from entering the nasal cavity and to allow the medication to flow in properly, occlude one nostril with your finger.

Insert the atomizer tip into the open nostril.
• Instruct the patient to inhale, and as he does so, squeeze the atomizer once, quickly and firmly. Use just enough force to coat the inside of the patient's nose with medication.
• If ordered, spray the nostril again. Then, repeat the procedure in the other nostril.
• Instruct the patient to keep his head tilted back for several minutes and to breathe slowly through his nose so the medication has time to work. Tell him not to blow his nose.
• Rinse the atomizer tip with warm water to prevent contamination of the medication with nasal secretions.

Continued

Nasal spray

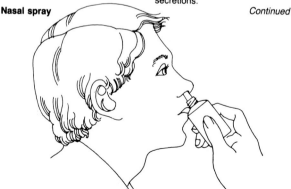

Instilling Nasal Medications
Continued

To use a nasal aerosol:
• Instruct the patient to clear his nostrils by gently blowing his nose.
• Insert the medication cartridge according to the manufacturer's directions.
• Shake the aerosol well immediately before each use, and remove the protective cap from the adapter tip.
• Hold the aerosol between your thumb and index finger, with your index finger on top of the medication cartridge.
• Tilt the patient's head back, and carefully insert the adapter tip in one nostril, while occluding the other nostril with your finger.
• Press the adapter and cartridge together firmly to release one measured dose of medication.
• Shake the aerosol, and repeat the procedure to instill medication into the other nostril.

Special considerations
Caution him against using nasal medications longer than prescribed, because they may cause a rebound effect that worsens the condition. During rebound, the medication loses its effectiveness and relaxes the vessels in the nasal turbinates, producing a stuffiness that can be relieved only by discontinuing the medication.

ORAL AND DERMATOMUCOSAL MEDICATIONS

Nasal aerosol

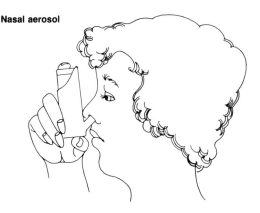

Administering Mouth and Throat Medications

Pharyngeal sprays, mouthwashes, and lozenges (troches) have a local action on the patient's mouth and throat.

To apply mouth or throat sprays:
• Make sure the medication's warmed.
• Seat your patient upright, and explain the procedure to him.
• Ask the patient to open his mouth. If you're administering an anesthetic, invert a teaspoon's bowl over the patient's tongue *before* you spray. Ask him to hold it. This will keep his tongue from getting numb. It will also help you see the irritated throat area. Instruct the patient to avoid inhaling as the medication's being administered.
• Hold the spray pump's nozzle just *outside* the patient's mouth, and direct the medication toward his throat. If you're using an atomizer, insert its tip just *inside* the patient's mouth, and direct the medication toward the back of his throat.

Squeeze the container quickly and firmly, using enough force to propel the spray to the inflamed throat tissues. Caution the patient not to swallow immediately, so the medication can run down his throat and coat the mucous membranes.

To administer a mouthwash or gargle:
• Warm the solution by immersing its container in hot water.
• If you're using the solution as a mouthwash, instruct him to swish ⅛ to ½ cup (30 to 120 ml) of the solution around in his mouth, especially over his teeth and gums. Warn him not to swallow it. Instead, instruct him to spit it into the emesis basin.
• If you're using the solution as a gargle, seat your patient upright, with his head erect or tilted back slightly. Ask him to take a deep breath. Then, give him ⅛ cup of the solution, and tell him to hold it in his mouth. Then, instruct him to exhale slowly, to create the gargling action. Tell him to spit the solution into the emesis basin.

To administer lozenges:
• If you're administering a lozenge, instruct the patient not to chew it. Instead, tell him to keep it in his mouth until it dissolves.

Special considerations
• If you've administered an anesthetic spray, warn your patient not to eat or drink anything for at least 1 hour afterward. The anesthetic will inhibit his gag reflex and increase the risk of aspiration.
• If the doctor's ordered a medication such as lidocaine hydrochloride (Xylocaine Viscous*), he may want you to instruct the patient to *swallow* the solution, so it coats and soothes irritated throat tissue.

*Available in the United States and Canada

Using Hand-held Oropharyngeal Inhalers

Hand-held inhalers include the metered-dose nebulizer, the turbo-inhaler, and the nasal inhaler. These devices deliver topical medications to the respiratory tract, producing both local and systemic effects. The mucosal lining of the respiratory tract absorbs the inhalant almost immediately. Examples of common inhalants are bronchodilators, used to facilitate mucous drainage, and mucolytics, which attain a high local concentration to liquefy tenacious bronchial secretions.

Use of a hand-held inhaler may be contraindicated in patients who can't form an airtight seal around the device, and in patients who lack the coordination or clear vision necessary to assemble a turbo-inhaler. Contraindications for specific inhalant drugs are also possible.

To use the metered-dose nebulizer:
• Remove the mouthpiece and cap from the bottle.
• Insert the bottle's metal stem into the small hole on the flattened mouthpiece portion. Then, turn the bottle upside down.
• Have the patient exhale, and then place the mouthpiece in his mouth and tell him to close his lips around it.
• Instruct him to inhale slowly as you firmly push the bottle down against the mouthpiece once. To draw the medication into his

Metered-dose nebulizer

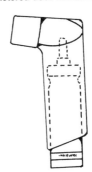

ORAL AND DERMATOMUCOSAL MEDICATIONS

lungs, tell him to continue inhaling until his lungs feel full.
• Remove the mouthpiece from the patient's mouth, and tell him to hold his breath for several seconds to allow the medication to reach the alveoli. Then, instruct him to exhale slowly through pursed lips to keep the distal bronchioles open, allowing increased absorption and diffusion of the drug and better gas exchange.
• Have the patient gargle with normal saline solution, if desired, to remove medication from the mouth and back of the throat. (The lungs retain only about 10% of the inhalant; most of the remainder is exhaled, but substan-

Continued

Using Hand-held Oropharyngeal Inhalers
Continued

Turbo-inhaler

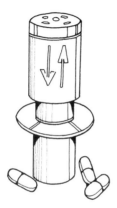

tial amounts may remain in the oropharynx.)
To use a turbo-inhaler:
• Hold the mouthpiece in one hand, and with the other hand slide the sleeve away from the mouthpiece as far as it will go.
• Unscrew the tip of the mouthpiece by turning it counterclockwise.
• Firmly press the colored portion of the medication capsule into the propeller stem of the mouthpiece.
• Screw the inhaler together again securely.
• Holding the inhaler with the mouthpiece at the bottom, slide the sleeve all the way down and then up again to puncture the capsule and release the medication. Do this only once.
• Have the patient exhale completely and tilt his head back. Then, instruct him to place the mouthpiece in his mouth, close his lips around it, and inhale once, quickly and deeply, through the mouthpiece.
• Tell the patient to hold his breath for several seconds to allow the medication to reach the alveoli. (Instruct him not to exhale through the mouthpiece.)
• Remove the inhaler from the patient's mouth, and tell him to exhale as much air as possible.
• Repeat the procedure until all the medication in the device is inhaled.
• Have the patient gargle with normal saline solution, if desired, to remove medication from the mouth and back of the throat. Be sure to provide an emesis basin if needed.
To use a nasal inhaler:
• Have the patient blow his nose to clear his nostrils.
• Insert the medication cartridge in the adapter. (When inserting a refill cartridge, first remove the protective cap from the stem.)
• Shake the inhaler well, and remove the protective cap.

Continued

Using Hand-held Oropharyngeal Inhalers
Continued

Nasal inhaler

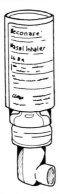

• Hold the inhaler with your index finger on top of the cartridge and your thumb under the nasal adapter. The adapter tip should be pointing toward the patient.
• Have the patient tilt his head back. Then, tell him to place the adapter tip into one nostril, while occluding the other nostril with his finger.

• Instruct the patient to inhale gently as he presses the adapter and the cartridge together firmly to release a measured medication dose. *Note:* Follow manufacturer's instructions. Some medications shouldn't be inhaled during administration.
• Tell the patient to remove the inhaler from his nostril and to exhale through his mouth.
• Shake the inhaler, and have the patient repeat the procedure in the other nostril.
• Have the patient gargle with normal saline solution to remove medication from the mouth and throat, if desired.

Special considerations
• When using a turbo-inhaler or a nasal inhaler, make sure the pressurized cartridge isn't punctured or incinerated. Store the medication cartridge below 120° F. (48.9° C.).
• If you're using a turbo-inhaler, keep the medication capsules wrapped until needed to keep them from deteriorating.

ORAL AND DERMATOMUCOSAL MEDICATIONS

Administering IPPB Therapy

Intermittent positive-pressure breathing (IPPB) delivers room air or oxygen into the lungs at a pressure higher than atmospheric pressure. This delivery ceases when pressure in the mouth or in the breathing circuit tube rises to a predetermined positive pressure. Although IPPB was once the mainstay of pulmonary therapy, its routine use is currently controversial.

However, proponents believe that IPPB treatments expand lung volumes more fully and promote an effective cough; deliver aerosolized medications deeper into the air passages; decrease the work of breathing; and assist in the mobilization of secretions.

IPPB treatment is contraindicated in uncompensated pneumothorax and tracheoesophageal fistula. Active hemoptysis or recent gastric surgery may also contraindicate this therapy.

Consider the patient who needs prolonged nebulization therapy several times a day. To help him, the doctor may order intermittent positive pressure breathing (IPPB) therapy. Briefly, here's how it works:

First, set the ventilator for the prescribed pressure. Connect either a mouthpiece or a mask to the ventilator, and ask the patient to inhale through it. The ventilator will automatically force a flow of nebulized medication into the patient's lungs until the preset pressure is reached. Then, when the machine shuts off, tell the patient to remove the mouthpiece or mask and exhale completely. Repeat the process for 10 or 15 minutes each session, as ordered.

After treatment, the patient may have episodes of coughing. Assure him that coughing is both normal and beneficial.

Whenever giving IPPB therapy, stay alert for these danger signs:
• sudden drop in blood pressure accompanied by increased heart rate, possibly indicating decreased venous return to heart
• nausea
• tremors or dizziness
• rapid, shallow respirations, possibly indicating respiratory alkalosis
• distended abdomen caused by gastric insufflation
• thickening of secretions caused by inadequate humidification

Evaluating Common Oxygen Delivery Systems

Oxygen, a potent drug, can be administered by cannula (nasal prongs), catheter, or mask to prevent or reverse hypoxia and improve tissue oxygenation. To compare oxygen delivery systems, read the information below.

NASAL CANNULA
(Low-flow system)

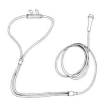

Advantages
- Comfortable; easily tolerated
- Nasal prongs can be shaped to fit facial contour.
- Effective for delivering low oxygen concentrations
- Allows freedom of movement; doesn't impede eating or talking
- Inexpensive; disposable
- Can provide continuous positive airway pressure for infants and children

SIMPLE FACE MASK
(Low-flow system)

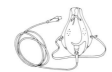

Advantages
- Effectively delivers high oxygen concentrations
- Humidification can be enhanced by using large-bore tubing and aerosol mask.
- Doesn't dry mucous membranes of nose and mouth

PARTIAL REBREATHER MASK
(Low-flow system)

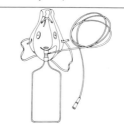

Advantages
- Oxygen reservoir bag lets pa-
Continued

Evaluating Common Oxygen Delivery Systems
Continued

PARTIAL REBREATHER MASK
Continued

tient rebreathe exhaled air from the trachea and bronchi. This increases his fraction of inspired oxygen concentration (FIO_2).
• Safety valve allows inhalation of room air if oxygen source fails.
• Effectively delivers high oxygen concentrations
• Easily humidifies oxygen
• Doesn't dry mucous membranes
• Can be converted to a nonrebreather mask, if necessary

NONREBREATHER MASK
(Low-flow system)

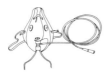

Advantages
• Delivers the highest possible oxygen concentration (60% to 90%) short of intubation and mechanical ventilation

• Effective for short-term therapy
• Doesn't dry mucous membranes
• Can be converted to a partial rebreather mask, if necessary

VENTURI MASK
(High-flow system)

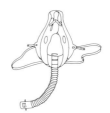

Advantages
• Delivers exact oxygen concentration despite patient's respiratory pattern or if flowmeter knob is bumped
• Diluter jets can be changed, or dial-turned, to change oxygen concentration
• Doesn't dry mucous membranes
• Can be used to deliver humidity or aerosol therapy

ORAL AND DERMATOMUCOSAL MEDICATIONS

Administering Medications Endotracheally

Administering medications directly into an endotracheal tube permits their absorption into the circulation via the alveoli. Endotracheal medication administration may be performed during cardiopulmonary resuscitation or when venous access is limited and an endotracheal tube's in place.

Medications that may be administered by the endotracheal route include epinephrine, atropine, lidocaine, naloxone, and metaraminol. Medications not recommended for endotracheal administration include calcium, sodium bicarbonate, and bretylium.

Follow these guidelines when administering medications endotracheally:

• Prepare the medication, preferably using a prefilled syringe containing the appropriate dose. If a prefilled syringe isn't available, use a standard 5- to 10-ml syringe with the needle or catheter securely attached. Use a syringe with the longest needle or catheter available to deliver the drug as deeply as possible.

• Check to see that the endotracheal tube's correctly placed and that the patient's positioned supine, with his head level with or higher than his trunk.

• Attach a positive-pressure oxygen delivery device, such as an Ambu bag, to the endotracheal tube. Quickly compress the bag

three to five times, then remove the device.

• Inject the medication quickly and deeply into the endotracheal tube. To prevent medication reflux, briefly place your thumb over the tube.

• After administering the medication, reattach the Ambu bag to the endotracheal tube and quickly compress it three to five times to help oxygenate the patient and distribute the medication.

Special considerations

• Unlike intracardiac medication administration, endotracheal administration doesn't interrupt basic life-support measures.

• To help prevent infection, keep the procedure as sterile as possible.

• As ordered, administer the same medication dose for endotracheal administration as you would for I.V. administration.

• If the patient doesn't respond to the first medication dose, repeat the dose. However, onset of action varies, depending on the medication and technique used and on the presence of conditions such as oxygen toxicity or adult respiratory distress syndrome.

• Medications administered endotracheally may have a longer duration of action compared to those administered I.V. Consequently, repeated doses and/or continuous infusion therapy may need to be readjusted. Carefully monitor the patient for signs and symptoms of toxicity.

ORAL AND DERMATOMUCOSAL MEDICATIONS

Injection Tips

Of all the ways to give medications, injection is the most hazardous. If you inject a medication incorrectly, you may damage the patient's nerves, tissue, or blood vessels or introduce bacteria into his system. To avoid complications, follow these guidelines:

• Select the site carefully to avoid major nerves and blood vessels.
• Don't select areas that have lesions, inflammation, hair, or birthmarks.
• Use only sterile needles and syringes.
• Make sure the needle you select is the proper length for the injection and the patient's body size.
• Always check for blood backflow before injecting. For intradermal, subcutaneous, and intramuscular injections, you don't want a backflow. If you notice blood in the syringe barrel, remove the needle and replace it with a new one. Then select another site and try again. (Be sure to discard both needles afterward.) For intravenous injections, you must get a blood backflow before proceeding. This tells you the needle's in the vein.
• Make sure someone's nearby to help restrain the patient, if necessary.
• Establish a site rotation plan for the patient who'll undergo repeated injections. Record the plan on his Kardex, so everyone can refer to it.

Major Injection Routes

INTRADERMAL

Site
Skin
Common needle sizes
26G × ⅜″ (0.95 cm)
Common dosage
0.1 ml
Dosage range
0.01 to 0.1 ml

SUBCUTANEOUS

Site
Subcutaneous fat beneath layers of skin
Common needle sizes
25G to 27G × ½″ to 1″ (1.27 to 2.54 cm)
Common dosage
0.5 ml
Dosage range
0.5 to 2 ml

Continued

Major Injection Routes
Continued

INTRAMUSCULAR

Site
Mid-deltoid
Common needle sizes
23G to 25G × ⅝" to 1" (1.59 to 2.54 cm)
Common dosage
0.5 ml
Dosage range
0.5 to 2 ml
Site
Gluteus medius (dorsogluteal)
Common needle sizes
20G to 23G × 1½" to 3" (3.81 to 7.62 cm)
Common dosage
2 to 4 ml
Dosage range
1 to 5 ml
Site
Gluteus medius and minimus (ventrogluteal)
Common needle sizes
20G to 23G × 1½" to 3" (3.81 to 7.62 cm)
Common dosage
1 to 4 ml
Dosage range
1 to 5 ml
Site
Vastus lateralis (preferred site for infants and children)

Common needle sizes
Infants and children:
22G to 25G × ⅝" to 1" (1.59 to 2.54 cm)
Adults:
20G to 23G × 1½" (3.81 cm)
Common dosage
1 to 4 ml
Dosage and range
1 to 5 ml
Site
Rectus femoris (alternate site for infants)
Common needle sizes
22G to 25G × ½" to 1" (1.27 to 2.54 cm)
Common dosage
1 to 2 ml
Dosage range
1 to 3 ml

INTRAVENOUS

Site
Basilic and cephalic veins
Common needle sizes
25G × ⅝" (1.59 cm) for slow injections; 19G to 23G × 1" to 1½" (2.54 to 3.81 cm)
Common dosage
1 to 10 ml
Dosage range
0.5 to 50 ml

Using a Cartridge Injection System

A cartridge injection system, such as the Tubex or Carpuject, is a convenient, easy-to-use injection method that facilitates both accuracy and sterility. It consists of a metal (usually chrome-plated brass) or plastic cartridge holder syringe and a prefilled medication cartridge with needle attached. In this system, the medication is premixed and premeasured, which saves time and helps ensure an exact dose. Because it's a closed system, the medication remains sealed in the cartridge until the injection's administered, maintaining sterility.

This system does have a drawback—not all drugs come in cartridge form. Compatible drugs can be added to partially filled cartridges.

To use a metal cartridge injection syringe (Tubex):

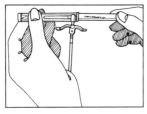

• Swing the handle section down, so it hangs at a right angle to the barrel, as shown here. Then, slide the sterile cartridge-needle unit—

needle-end first—into the barrel. Holding the metal syringe barrel, swing the plunger rod back into place, and engage the plunger into the cartridge by turning the plunger clockwise until you hear a click at the front of the syringe. Both ends of the cartridge-needle unit should be engaged in the syringe before injection.

• After the injection, rest the syringe against the palm of one hand, needle pointing up. Holding the rubber sheath covering the needle between the thumb and forefinger of the other hand, slide it over the needle tip. Shake the syringe gently to allow gravity to cause the sheath to fall back into position. Pull down on the bottom of the sheath to cover the needle completely.

• Hold the glass cartridge with one hand, and with the other hand rotate the plunger rod counterclockwise to disengage it. Pull the plunger rod back, and open the syringe. Be careful that you don't pull back on the plunger rod before disengaging it, or it will jam.

• Disengage the glass cartridge by rotating it counterclockwise, and remove it from the syringe. Discard the cartridge and sheath-covered needle according to institution policy.

Continued

PARENTERAL MEDICATIONS

Using a Cartridge Injection System
Continued

To use a plastic cartridge injection syringe (Carpuject):

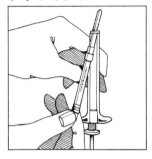

• Grasp the syringe barrel with the open side facing you, and pull back the plunger rod as far as possible.
• Disengage the locking screw by turning it counterclockwise.
• Insert the cartridge-needle unit—needle-end first—into the open side of the barrel. Advance and engage the locking screw, and turn it clockwise beyond its initial resistance until it will no longer rotate. Advance the plunger rod and screw clockwise onto the threaded insert in the rubber plunger.

• After the injection, replace the sheath. Disengage the plunger rod from the plunger by rotating it counterclockwise and pulling it back as far as possible.
• Disengage the locking screw by rotating it counterclockwise. Turn the syringe over, and remove the cartridge-needle unit. Discard the unit according to institution policy.
To add a compatible medication to a partially filled cartridge:
• Hold the cartridge with the needle end up. Pull back the plunger rod so the rubber piston surface in contact with the medication is set at the 2.5-ml mark.
• Wipe the diaphragm of the vial containing the compatible medication with an alcohol sponge.
• Insert the needle into the single-dose vial. Depress the plunger rod to inject into the vial an amount of air equal to the prescribed medication amount to be withdrawn from the vial. Pull the rod back to withdraw the medication.
• Remove the needle from the vial, expel excess air, and replace the rubber sheath.
• Proceed to the patient's room to give the injection. Discard the equipment according to institution policy.

Combining Drugs in a Syringe

Combining two drugs in one syringe avoids the discomfort of two separate injections. Usually, drugs can be mixed in a syringe in one of three ways. They may be combined from two multidose vials (regular and long-acting insulin, for example, can be combined this way). They can also be combined from one multidose vial and one ampul, or from two ampuls.

Such combinations are contraindicated when the drugs aren't compatible or when the combined doses exceed the amount of solution that can be absorbed from a single injection site.

To mix drugs from two multidose vials:
• Using an alcohol sponge, wipe the rubber stopper on the first vial. This decreases the possibility of introducing microorganisms into the medication as you insert the needle into the vial.
• Pull back the syringe plunger until the volume of air drawn into the syringe equals the volume to be withdrawn from the drug vial.
• Without inverting the vial, insert the needle into the top of the vial, making sure that the bevel's tip doesn't touch the solution. Inject the air into the vial and withdraw

the needle. This replaces air in the vial to prevent creation of a partial vacuum when the drug is withdrawn.
• Repeat the above steps for the second vial. Then, after injecting the air into the second vial, invert the vial, withdraw the prescribed dose, and then withdraw the needle.
• Wipe the rubber stopper of the first vial again and insert the needle, taking care not to depress the plunger. Invert the vial, withdraw the prescribed dose, and then withdraw the needle.
To mix drugs from one multidose vial and one ampul:
• Using an alcohol sponge, clean the vial's rubber stopper.
• Pull back on the syringe plunger until the volume of air drawn into the syringe equals the volume to be withdrawn from the drug vial.
• Insert the needle into the top of the vial and inject the air. Then, invert the vial and withdraw the prescribed dose. Put the sterile needle cover over the needle.

Wrap the ampul neck with sterile gauze or an alcohol sponge to protect yourself from injury in case the glass splinters. Break open the ampul, directing the force away from you.

Continued

PARENTERAL MEDICATIONS

Combining Drugs in a Syringe
Continued

• If desired, switch to a filter needle at this point to filter out any glass splinters.
• Insert the needle into the ampul. Be careful not to touch the outside of the ampul with the needle. Draw the correct dose into the syringe.
• If you switched to the filter needle, change back to a regular needle to administer the drugs.
To mix drugs from two ampuls:
• An opened ampul doesn't contain a vacuum. To mix drugs from two ampuls in a syringe, calculate the prescribed doses and open both ampuls, using aseptic technique. If desired, use a filter needle to draw up the drugs. Then, change to a regular needle to administer them.

Special considerations
• Never combine two drugs if you're unsure of their compatibility. When in doubt, administer two separate injections. Never try to combine more than two drugs.
• Insert the needle through the vial's rubber stopper at a slight angle, bevel up, and exert slight lateral pressure. This way you won't cut a piece of rubber out of the stopper, which can then be pushed into the vial.
• When mixing drugs from multidose vials, be careful not to contaminate the second drug with the first. Ideally, the needle should be changed after drawing the first medication into the syringe. This isn't always possible, because many disposable syringes don't have removable needles. Insulin is one of the few drugs that still comes in multidose vials. Be careful when mixing regular and long-acting insulin. Draw up the regular insulin first to avoid contamination by the long-acting suspension. If a minute amount of regular insulin accidentally mixes with the long-acting insulin, it won't appreciably change the effect of the long-acting insulin. Because the issue of which insulin should be drawn up first is controversial, check institution policy regarding this matter.
• With a cartridge injection system and a multidose vial, use a separate needle and syringe to inject the air into the multidose vial. This prevents possible contamination of the multidose vial by the cartridge injection system.

Drugs Combined in a Syringe: Compatibility Table

	atropine	butorphanol	chlorpromazine	codeine	diazepam	glycopyrrolate	hydromorphone	hydroxyzine	meperidine	morphine	nalbuphine	pentobarbital	phenobarbital	promethazine	scopolamine	secobarbital	sodium bicarbonate	thiopental
atropine		●	▽	○	▼	●	○	▽	▽	▽	●	▽	○	▽	▽	○	▼	○
butorphanol	●		▽	○	▼	●	○	●	○	○	○	▼	▼	●	●	▼	○	▼
chlorpromazine	▽	▽		○	▼	●	○	▼	▽	▽	○	▼	▼	▽	▽	▼	○	▼
codeine	○	○	○		▼	●	○	▽	○	○	○	▼	○	○	○	○	▼	○
diazepam	▼	▼	▼	▼		▼	▼	▼	▼	▼	▼	▼	▼	▼	▼	▼	▼	▼
glycopyrrolate	●	●	●	●	▼		●	●	●	●	●	○	●	●	▼	○	○	○
hydromorphone	○	○	○	○	▼	●		○	○	○	●	○	○	○	○	○	▼	▼
hydroxyzine	▽	●	▼	▽	▼	●	○		▽	▽	●	▼	▼	▼	▽	▽	○	○
meperidine	▽	○	▽	○	▼	●	○	▽		○	○	▽	▼	▽	○	▼	▽	▼
morphine	▽	○	▽	○	▼	●	○	▽	○		▼	■	●	▼	▽	○	▼	▼
nalbuphine	●	○	○	○	▼	●	●	●	○	▼		▼	○	●	●	○	○	○
pentobarbital	▽	▼	▼	▼	▼	○	○	▼	▽	■	▼		○	▼	▽	○	■	▽
phenobarbital	○	▼	▼	○	▼	●	○	▼	▼	●	○	○		▼	○	○	○	●
promethazine	▽	●	▽	○	▼	●	○	▼	▽	▼	●	▼	▼		▽	○	○	■
scopolamine	▽	●	▽	○	▼	▼	○	▽	○	▽	●	▽	○	▽		▼	▼	●
secobarbital	○	▼	▼	○	▼	○	○	▽	▼	○	○	○	○	○	▼		○	○
sodium bicarbonate	▼	○	○	▼	▼	○	▼	○	▽	▼	○	■	○	○	▼	○		▼
thiopental	○	▼	▼	○	▼	○	▼	○	▼	▼	○	▽	●	■	●	○	▼	

KEY

- ● compatible
- ▼ not compatible
- ▽ provisionally compatible; use within 15 minutes of preparation
- ○ no available data on compatibility
- ■ conflicting reports on compatibility; mixing not recommended

Intradermal Injection Sites

If your patient needs an intradermal injection, you'll probably give it in her ventral forearm. But if her arms are burned or irritated, you could substitute her upper chest or a shoulder blade. The sites you can use are shown here. The skin in these areas is lightly pigmented, thinly keratinized, and usually hairless. These qualities make it easy to observe reactions to the injection. *Note:* Don't expect *immediate results*. The capillaries of the dermis have a slower absorption rate than subcutaneous tissue or muscle.

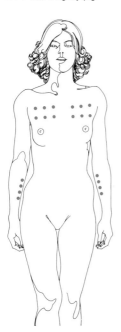
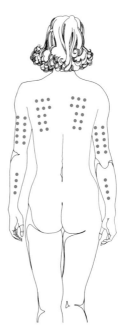

Administering Intradermal Medications

The doctor orders intradermal medications when he wants to produce a local effect or to give skin tests for allergy or anergy testing. As ordered, use a tuberculin syringe with a 26G or 27G needle.

Follow these guidelines when administering intradermal medications:

• The ventral forearm, perhaps the most commonly used intradermal injection site, allows easy access and lacks hair. Cleanse the area with an alcohol swab, applying pressure and using a circular motion. *Important:* Never use a disinfectant, such as povidone-iodine (Betadine), which will discolor the skin. And don't rub so hard you cause irritation. Either action could hinder the test reading.

Allow the skin to dry thoroughly. If you inject the needle while the skin's wet, you may accidentally introduce antiseptic into the dermis.

• Hold the patient's forearm in one hand, and stretch his skin with your thumb. Then, with your other hand, hold the syringe between your thumb and forefinger and rest the plunger against your palm's heel. Expel any air in the needle.

• Position the syringe so that the needle's almost flat against the patient's skin (at approximately a 15° angle). Make sure the needle's bevel faces upward.

• Insert the needle by pressing it against the skin until you meet resistance. Then, advance it through the epidermis so that you can see its point through the skin. Stop when it rests ⅛" (3 mm) below the skin's surface, between the epidermis and the dermal layers.

• Now inject the medication as slowly and gently as possible. Expect to feel some resistance—this means that the needle's properly placed. If the plunger moves freely, you've inserted it too deeply. When you've finished injecting the medication, leave the needle in place momentarily. Watch for a small white bleb or wheal to form.

• When the bleb or wheal appears, withdraw the needle and apply gentle pressure to the site. Don't massage it, because doing so may interfere with test results.

How to Perform and Interpret the Mantoux (PPD) Test for Tuberculosis

• Check the label of the PPD vial for drug strength and expiration date. (PPD is available in three strengths, containing 1, 5, or 250 tuberculin units. The intermediate strength, containing 5 tuberculin units, is the one most often used for diagnostic testing.)

• Use an easy-to-read tuberculin syringe with a 25G needle.

• After you draw the PPD into the syringe, administer it within 5 minutes (it can be absorbed by glass and plastic).

• After cleansing the site with alcohol, allow the skin to dry and then inject the PPD in the upper third of the patient's ventral forearm, just beneath the skin's surface (intradermal injection). Be sure the needle bevel is facing up.

• A wheal—a pale elevation of skin—6 to 10 mm in diameter should appear immediately.

• If no wheal forms, the injection may have been too deep. Reinject the PPD at a site at least 2″ (5 cm) from the first site, or on the other arm.

• To interpret the skin test, measure the area of induration (hardening or thickening of tissues)

at 48 and 72 hours. (*Note:* Erythema isn't generally considered evidence of an active or dormant infection.)

An induration of 10 mm or greater indicates a significant reaction. (This was formerly called a positive reaction.) Significance of a reaction is determined not only by the size of the reaction but by circumstances. For example, a reaction of 5 mm or more may be considered significant in a person who has an immediate family member with tuberculosis.

• Record results for attending doctor.

Note: A significant PPD reaction usually results in patients previously vaccinated with bacille Calmette-Guérin (BCG) vaccine. If you know a patient has received the BCG vaccine, don't administer the PPD test. Also, a false-negative reaction can occur in an anergic patient (who can't react to any skin tests) or in an immunosuppressed patient.

Tuberculosis diagnosis must be confirmed by chest X-ray and/or positive sputum smear.

PARENTERAL MEDICATIONS

Source: Centers for Disease Control criteria, and American Thoracic Surgeons Society statement on tuberculosis skin test reactions, August 1981

Subcutaneous Injection Sites

Subcutaneous injection sites (shown by dotted areas) include the fat pads on the abdomen, upper hips, upper back, and lateral upper arms and thighs. For subcutaneous injections administered regularly, rotate sites. Choose one injection site in one area, move to a corresponding injection site in the next area, and so on. When returning to an area, choose a new site in that area.

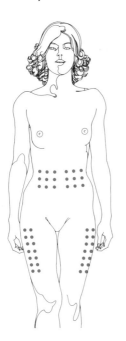
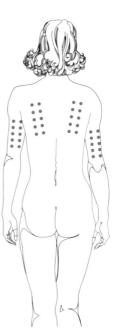

Administering Subcutaneous Injections

Injection into the adipose tissues (fatty layer) beneath the skin delivers a drug into the bloodstream more rapidly than oral administration. Subcutaneous injection allows slower, more sustained drug administration than intramuscular injection; it also causes minimal tissue trauma and carries little risk of striking large blood vessels and nerves.

Absorbed mainly through the capillaries, drugs recommended for subcutaneous injection are nonirritating aqueous solutions and suspensions contained in fluid volumes of 0.5 to 2.0 ml. They're injected through a relatively short needle, using meticulous sterile technique.

The most common subcutaneous injection sites include the outer aspect of the upper arm, anterior thigh, loose tissue of the lower abdomen, buttocks, and upper back. Injection is contraindicated in sites that are inflamed, edematous, scarred, or covered with moles, birthmarks, or other lesions.

Follow these guidelines when administering subcutaneous injections:

• Select a needle of the right gauge and length. An average adult patient requires a 25G ⅝″ needle; an infant, a child, or an elderly or thin patient, a 25G to 27G ½″ needle.

• Select an appropriate injection site. Rotate sites according to a planned schedule for patients who require repeated injections. Use different areas of the body unless contraindicated by the specific drug (heparin, for example, can be injected only in certain sites).

• Cleanse the injection site with a sterile alcohol sponge. Allow the skin to dry before injecting the drug to avoid a stinging sensation from introducing alcohol into subcutaneous tissues.

• Loosen the protective needle sheath.

• With your nondominant hand, grasp the skin around the injection site firmly to elevate the subcutaneous tissue, forming a 1″ (2.5-cm) fat fold.

• Holding the syringe in your dominant hand, insert the loosened needle sheath between the fourth and fifth fingers of your other hand, still pinching the skin around the injection site. Pull back the syringe with your dominant hand to uncover the needle by grasping the syringe like a pencil.

• Position the needle with its bevel up.

• Insert the needle at a 45° or 90° angle to the skin surface, depending on the amount of subcuta-

Continued

Administering Subcutaneous Injections
Continued

neous tissue at the site and the needle length. Some medications, such as heparin, should always be injected at a 90° angle.
• Insert the needle quickly, in one motion. Release the patient's skin to avoid injecting into compressed tissue and irritating nerve fibers.
• Pull back the plunger slightly to aspirate for blood return. If none appears, begin injecting the drug slowly. If blood appears upon aspiration, withdraw the needle, prepare another syringe, and repeat the procedure.
• After injection, remove the needle gently but quickly at the same angle used for insertion.

• Cover the site with an alcohol sponge, and massage the site gently (unless you have injected a drug that contraindicates massage, such as heparin) to distribute the drug and facilitate absorption.
• Remove the sponge, and check the injection site for bleeding or bruising.
Special considerations
• Concentrated or irritating solutions may cause sterile abscesses to form. A natural immune response, this complication can be minimized by rotating injection sites. Repeated injections in the same site can cause lipodystrophy.

Subcutaneous Medication Administration

The absorption of medication given by any parenteral route is chiefly influenced by blood flow. Since subcutaneous tissue has minimal blood flow, the absorption rate is usually slow. But a few medications, such as heparin, defy this rule; they're absorbed through the subcutaneous tissue as rapidly as they are through intramuscular tissue.

Here are some other ways absorption is affected:

• The trauma of injection releases histamine into subcutaneous tissue, which decreases blood flow and *slows* absorption.
• Physical exertion increases blood flow in subcutaneous tissue, in turn speeding up the absorption rate.
• Normal connective tissue prevents medication from spreading indiscriminately and slows the absorption rate.

Administering Heparin Injections

To inject heparin, follow the usual procedure for any subcutaneous injection, except for these considerations:
• Use a 25G or 26G ½″ needle.
• The preferred site for heparin injections is the lower abdominal fat pad, 2″ (5 cm) beneath the umbilicus, from iliac crest to crest (see illustration). Injecting heparin into this area, which isn't involved in muscular activity, reduces the risk of local capillary bleeding. Always rotate the sites from one side to the other.
• Don't administer any injections within 2″ of a scar, a bruise, or the umbilicus.

• Pinch a ½″ (1.3 cm) fold of tissue between your thumb and forefinger, and insert the needle into the fold at a 90° angle. Using this technique will minimize heparin's irritating qualities.
• Don't aspirate to check for blood return because this may cause bleeding into the tissues at the site.
• Don't rub or massage the site after the injection. Rubbing can cause localized minute hemorrhages or bruises.
• If the patient bruises easily, apply ice to the site for the first 5 minutes after the injection to minimize local hemorrhage.

PARENTERAL MEDICATIONS

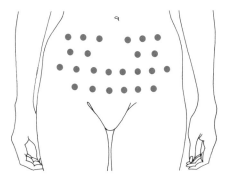

Subcutaneous Injections: What to Tell the Diabetic Patient

Be sure to teach your diabetic patient how to rotate his injection sites systematically and mix his insulin (if necessary). Explain to him that if he fails to rotate the injection site, he could experience any of the following tissue complications:

• *Atrophy* (subcutaneous fat loss). A small dimple or depression will form at the injection site, interfering with absorption. This can scar or desensitize the area.

• *Hypertrophy* (thickening of the subcutaneous tissue). The skin around the injection site will appear lumpy, hard, or spongy. This condition also interferes with absorption and can scar or desensitize the area. (Hypertrophy may also be caused by delivering cold insulin.)

• *Unabsorbed insulin deposits.* The patient will show signs of hyperglycemia.

If he suddenly becomes more active or traumatizes the deposit, his subcutaneous circulation will increase, in turn increasing absorption and causing hypoglycemia.

If your patient must combine insulins in a syringe, caution him to make sure the insulin types are compatible. Regular insulin can be mixed with *all* types. Prompt insulin zinc suspension (Semilente) *cannot* be mixed with NPH insulin.

Suppose your diabetic patient must administer a combination of regular and NPH insulin. You must teach him how to draw them up in the same syringe without contaminating the vials. To do this, demonstrate the procedure by following these steps:

• Clean the top of both vials with alcohol.

• Draw air into the syringe in an amount equal to the prescribed dose of NPH insulin.

• Inject all the air into the NPH vial. Remove the syringe from the vial.

• Now, draw air into the syringe in an amount equal to the prescribed dose of regular insulin.

• Inject the air into the regular insulin vial. Then, invert the vial, and withdraw the prescribed dose of regular insulin.

• Before you remove the syringe, check for air bubbles in the syringe barrel. If any are present, lightly tap the syringe with your finger. Then, push up slightly on the plunger to force the air back into the vial. Make sure the syringe still contains the prescribed insulin dose. Then, withdraw the needle and syringe.

• Now, insert the needle into the NPH vial, and invert the vial. Withdraw the correct amount of NPH insulin.

CSII: A Blood Glucose Regulation System

Some patients with Type I diabetes mellitus can now benefit from an insulin infusion pump called the continuous subcutaneous insulin infuser (CSII). This device controls blood glucose levels more closely than traditional insulin injections. It mimics the normal pancreas by delivering at least a basal insulin amount continuously and by adjusting the insulin amount as needed. In addition, the patient can program it to deliver an insulin bolus before meals.

CSII consists of a computerized insulin pump and infusion set small enough to fit in a shirt pocket or hang from a belt. Typically, the pump has a display screen, control panel, alarm, battery chamber, motor, and insulin reservoir.

The patient fills the reservoir with regular insulin and programs the basal rates and bolus doses for the pump. A special battery fits into the back of the pump and runs its motor. The pump primes the infusion set, which is connected to the insulin reservoir. Insulin travels through the infusion set tubing to a subcutaneous needle that's taped in place after priming.

Your job is to reinforce this teaching, answer the patient's questions about his treatment, and assess his self-care skills and response to treatment. Here are some tips to make this easier.

• Ask the patient to report his blood glucose levels before meals and at bedtime, the times when he administered boluses of insulin, and the amount of food he ate at meals.

• Document this information in the patient's chart. Also record any signs of *hypoglycemia* or *hyperglycemia.*

• Remind the patient to change the battery and recharge it according to instructions.

• Help the patient change and fill the insulin reservoir each day.

• Aid the patient in changing the infusion set at least every 2 days. He should select a new insertion site that's at least 1″ away from the old one.

Guide to Intramuscular Injection Sites

When you're giving an intramuscular injection, you have five basic sites to choose from. The absorption rate for each site is about the same. Intramuscular absorption is similar to, but more rapid than, subcutaneous absorption because of increased blood flow to the muscles. For example, aqueous medications are absorbed from a muscle site within 10 to 30 minutes, while it takes over 30 minutes from a subcutaneous site.

Keep in mind, however, that not all intramuscular medications take effect at the same speed. Study the following illustrations to determine which site is best for your patient.

Ventrogluteal

Used for all patients. Desirable because the site is not only relatively free of large nerves and fat tissue, but remote from rectum (which minimizes the risk of contamination).

Position patient on his back or side.

Deltoid

Seldom used because the muscle is small and can accommodate only small doses. It's also dangerously near the radial nerve.

Seat patient upright or have him lie flat, with his arms apart.

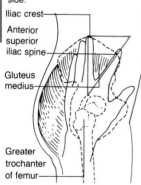

Iliac crest
Anterior superior iliac spine
Gluteus medius
Greater trochanter of femur

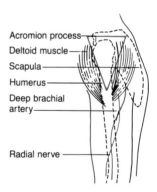

Acromion process
Deltoid muscle
Scapula
Humerus
Deep brachial artery
Radial nerve

Continued

Guide to Intramuscular Injection Sites
Continued

Vastus lateralis and rectus femoris
The vastus lateralis is used for all patients, especially children. The rectus femoris is most often used for self-injection because of its accessibility.

Position patient in bed either sitting up or lying flat.

Dorsogluteal
Commonly used for adults, but not for infants and children under age 3 because their dorsogluteal muscles aren't well developed.

Position patient flat on his stomach, with his toes pointed inward, and his arms apart and flexed toward his head.

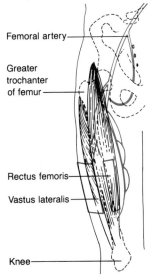

Femoral artery

Greater trochanter of femur

Rectus femoris

Vastus lateralis

Knee

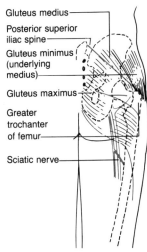

Gluteus medius

Posterior superior iliac spine

Gluteus minimus (underlying medius)

Gluteus maximus

Greater trochanter of femur

Sciatic nerve

Injecting Intramuscular Medications

Intramuscular (I.M.) injections deposit medication deep into muscle tissue, where a large network of blood vessels can absorb it readily and quickly. This administration route is preferred when rapid systemic action is desired and when relatively large doses (up to 5 ml in appropriate sites) are necessary. I.M. injections may be used for patients who can't take medication orally and for drugs changed by digestive juices. And because muscle tissue has few sensory nerves, I.M. injection allows less painful administration of irritating drugs.

The I.M. injection site must be chosen carefully, taking into account the patient's general physical status and the injection's purpose. I.M. injections should not be administered at inflamed, edematous, or irritated sites or those containing moles, birthmarks, scar tissue, or other lesions. I.M. injections may also be contraindicated in patients with impaired coagulation mechanisms and in patients with occlusive peripheral vascular disease, edema, and

shock, because these conditions impair peripheral absorption. I.M. injections require sterile technique to maintain muscle tissue integrity.

Follow these guidelines when administering I.M. injections:
• Draw up the prescribed amount of medication using the three-label check system—read the label as you select the medication, as you draw it up, and after you have completed drawing it up to assure correct dosage. Then draw about 0.2 cc of air into the syringe. When the syringe is inverted during injection, the air bubble rises to the syringe's plunger end and follows the medication into the injection site. The air clears the needle of medication and helps prevent leakage into subcutaneous tissue following injection by creating an air block that reduces reflux (tracking) along the needle path.
• Select an appropriate injection site. The gluteal muscles (gluteus medius and minimus, and the upper outer corner of the gluteus maximus) are most commonly used for

Continued

Injecting Intramuscular Medications
Continued

healthy adults, although the deltoid muscle may be used for a small-volume injection (2 ml or less). For infants and children, you may want to use the vastus lateralis thigh muscle because it's usually the best developed and contains no large nerves or blood vessels, minimizing the risk of serious injury. The rectus femoris muscle may also be used in infants but is usually contraindicated in adults.

• After locating the injection site, cleanse the skin at the site with an alcohol sponge. Then allow the skin to dry to prevent the alcohol from being introduced into the muscle tissue as the needle is inserted, causing pain or burning when it reaches the sensory nerve endings of subcutaneous tissue.

• With the thumb and index finger of your nondominant hand, gently stretch the skin of the injection site taut.

• Holding the syringe in your dominant hand, remove the needle sheath by slipping it between the free fingers of your nondominant hand and then drawing back the syringe.

• Position the syringe at a 90° angle to the skin surface, with the needle several inches from the skin. Then, quickly and firmly thrust the needle through the skin and subcutaneous tissue, deep into the muscle.

• Support the syringe with your nondominant hand, if desired. Pull back slightly on the plunger with your dominant hand to aspirate for blood. If no blood appears, place your thumb on the plunger rod and *slowly* inject the medication into the muscle. A slow, steady injection rate allows the muscle to distend gradually and accept the medication under minimal pressure. You should feel little or no resistance against the injection's force. The air bubble in the syringe should follow the medication into the injection site.

• If blood appears in the syringe on aspiration, the needle's in a blood vessel. If this occurs,
Continued

PARENTERAL MEDICATIONS

Injecting Intramuscular Medications
Continued

stop the injection, withdraw the needle, prepare another injection with new equipment, and inject another site. Don't inject the bloody solution.

• After the injection, gently but rapidly remove the needle at a 90° angle.

• Cover the injection site immediately with the used alcohol sponge, apply gentle pressure, and, unless contraindicated, massage the relaxed muscle to help distribute the drug and promote absorption.

• Remove the alcohol sponge and inspect the injection site for signs of active bleeding or bruising. If bleeding continues, apply pressure to the site; if bruising occurs, apply ice.

Special considerations

• Never use the gluteal muscles, which develop from walking, as the injection site for a child under age 3 or who has been walking for less than a year. Never inject sensitive muscles, especially those that twitch or tremble when you assess site landmarks and tissue depth with your fingertips. Injections in these trigger areas may cause sharp or referred pain,

such as the pain caused by nerve trauma.

• If the patient has experienced pain or emotional trauma from repeated injections, consider numbing the area before cleansing it by holding ice on it for several seconds. If you must inject more than 5 ml of solution, divide the solution and inject it at two separate sites.

• Always encourage the patient to relax the muscle you'll be injecting, because injections into tense muscles are more painful and may bleed more readily.

• Accidental injection of concentrated or irritating medications into subcutaneous tissue or other areas where it can't be fully absorbed can cause sterile abscesses. Such abscesses result from a natural immune response in which phagocytes attempt to remove the foreign matter.

• Failure to rotate sites in patients who require repeated injections can lead to deposits of unabsorbed drugs. Such deposits can reduce the desired pharmacologic effect and may lead to abscess formation or tissue fibrosis.

Using the Z-Track Method for Injection

1. If you're administering iron dextran complex (Imferon), you must vary the standard injection procedure by performing what's known as the Z-track method. It involves pulling the skin in such a way that the needle track is sealed off after the injection. Doing this minimizes subcutaneous irritation and discoloration. You'll inject the drug into the patient's buttock. To find out how, read on.
2. After drawing up 0.3 to 0.5 cc of air into the syringe, replace the needle with a sterile one that's 3″ (8 cm) long.

Pull the skin laterally away from the intended injection site. This will ensure proper entry of muscle tissue (bottom left illustration).
3. After cleansing the site, insert the needle, and inject the medication slowly (top right illustration).

When you've completed the injection, wait 10 seconds before you withdraw the needle. That way, you'll prevent medication seepage from the site.
4. Withdraw the needle and syringe. Now, allow the retracted skin to resume its normal position. This will effectively seal off the needle track (bottom right illustration).

Never massage the site or allow the patient to wear tight-fitting clothes. Otherwise, the medication could be forced into the subcutaneous tissue and cause irritation.

To increase the absorption rate, encourage physical activity; for example, walking. For subsequent injections, alternate buttocks.

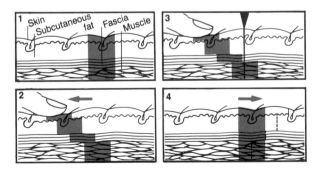

Reducing the Pain of Intramuscular Injections

You can reduce the pain of intra-muscular (I.M.) injections by following these tips:

• *Encourage your patient to relax the muscle you'll be injecting.* Injections into tense muscles cause more pain and bleeding than injections into relaxed muscles. (Give injections into the gluteal muscles while the patient lies face down with his toes pointed in, or on his side with the knee and hip of the upper leg flexed and anterior to the lower leg).

• *Avoid extrasensitive areas.* When you choose the injection site, roll the muscle mass under your fingers and look for twitching. This indicates an extrasensitive trigger area. Injections in this area may cause referred pain or a sharp pain as if the nerve were hit.

• *Wait until the skin antiseptic is dry.* If the antiseptic is still wet, it will cling to the needle, creating pain when it reaches the sensory nerves of the subcutaneous tissues.

• *Always use a new needle.* The point and bevel of the needle can be dulled when they pass through the rubber stoppers in vials. Unless you change the needle, the dulled or rough edge that results causes more friction and pain during

injection. Changing the needle also removes another source of pain—irritating medication that adheres to the outside of the needle when you draw the medication out of the vial.

• *Draw about 0.2 cc of air into the syringe.* This clears the needle bore of medication, which could leak out through the needle before or during insertion. When the needle is inverted for the injection, the air bubble rises to the plunger end of the syringe. Injecting this harmless air bubble reduces "tracking"—the leakage of medication from the needle injection path.

• *Dart the needle in rapidly and withdraw it rapidly to minimize puncture pain.*

• *Aspirate to be sure the needle isn't in a blood vessel.* Then, inject the medication slowly to allow it to spread into the tissue under less pressure.

• *Unless contraindicated, massage the relaxed muscle to distribute the medication better and increase its absorption.* This will reduce the pain caused by tissue stretching from a large-volume injection. (Physical exercise of the injected muscle serves the same purpose.)

I.V. Injection Methods

DIRECT (I.V. bolus)

To deliver drugs rapidly
Advantages
• Drug becomes effective immediately, because it's injected directly into patient's bloodstream.
• Absorption process more predictable than with other methods.
Disadvantages
• May cause speed shock
• More likely to irritate vein
• Increases risk of complications, including extravasation, systemic infection, air embolism

CONTINUOUS DRIP (primary line infusion)

To maintain delivery at a therapeutic level
Advantages
• Less irritating than bolus injection
• Requires less mixing and hanging than with intermittent method
• Easy to discontinue
Disadvantages
• Can be dangerous if I.V. flow rate isn't carefully monitored
• Many drugs don't remain stable for the length of time this method requires.
• Increases risk of complications, including extravasation, systemic infection, air embolism
• Mixing medications may cause incompatibility.

INTERMITTENT (additive set infusion)

To administer drugs mixed with diluent. May be infused intermittently over a period of time or as a one-time dose.
Advantages
• Administration time longer than bolus injection and shorter than continuous drip therapy
• Less likely to cause speed shock than bolus injection
• Less irritating to veins than bolus injection
Disadvantages
• Expensive
• Increased chance of contamination with frequent port use
• Mixing medications may cause incompatibility.
• Increases risk of complications, including extravasation, systemic infection, air embolism

PARENTERAL MEDICATIONS

I.V. Bolus (Push) Injections

The I.V. bolus injection method allows rapid intravenous administration of a drug. It may be used in an emergency to provide an immediate drug effect. It can also be used to achieve peak drug blood levels, to deliver drugs that can't be diluted or that can't be given intramuscularly because they're toxic to muscle tissue or because the patient has an impaired ability to absorb them.

The term bolus generally refers to a drug's concentration or amount. I.V. push is a technique for rapid intravenous injection.

Bolus medication doses may be injected directly into a vein or through an existing I.V. line. Medication administered by these methods takes effect rapidly. I.V. bolus injections are contraindicated when rapid drug administration could cause life-threatening complications or when the drug requires dilution.

To give direct injections:
• Select the largest vein suitable for an injection. The larger the vein, the more di-

luted the drug will become as it travels through it, minimizing vascular irritation.
• Apply a tourniquet above the injection site to distend the vein.
• Cleanse the injection site.
• If you're using the syringe's needle, insert it into the vein at a 30° angle with the bevel upwards. The bevel should reach ¼″ (0.6 cm) into the vein. If you're using a winged-tip needle, insert the needle (bevel up), tape the butterfly wings in place when you see blood return in the tubing, and attach the syringe containing the drug.
• Pull back on the plunger of the syringe and check for blood backflow, which indicates that the needle's in the vein.
• Remove the tourniquet and inject the drug at the appropriate rate.
• Pull back slightly on the syringe's plunger and check for blood backflow again. If blood appears, it indicates that the needle remained in place and all of the injected medication entered the vein.

Continued

I.V. Bolus (Push) Injections
Continued

• If you're using a winged-tip needle, flush the line with the normal saline solution from the second syringe to ensure delivery of all the medication into the vein.

• Withdraw the needle and apply pressure to the injection site with the sterile gauze pad for 3 minutes to prevent hematoma formation.

• Apply the adhesive bandage to the site after bleeding has stopped.

To give injections through an existing I.V. line:

• Check the compatibility of the medication with the I.V. solution.

• Close the flow clamp, wipe the injection port with a sterile alcohol sponge, and inject the drug as you would for direct injection.

• Open the flow clamp and readjust the flow rate.

• If the drug isn't compatible with the I.V. solution, flush the line with normal saline solution or bacteriostatic water before and after the injection.

Special considerations

• Because drugs administered by I.V. bolus or push injection are delivered directly into the circulatory system and can produce an immediate effect, signs of an acute allergic reaction or anaphylaxis can develop rapidly.

• Watch for signs of extravasation. If extravasation occurs, stop the injection, estimate the amount of infiltration, and notify the doctor.

• Before administering a bolus injection through an I.V. line that already contains a medication, evaluate the effects this action might cause. Remember—when you flush the line before and after giving the bolus injection, you're injecting a bolus dose of the original medication. In many cases, this won't affect the patient. However, if the I.V. line originally contained a drug such as a vasopressor, bolus injection could cause unwanted effects.

PARENTERAL MEDICATIONS

Continuous Drip Method

Various transfer devices can be used to add drugs to an I.V. solution. The common syringe and needle are used to draw up medications, reconstitute powdered drugs, and make transfers. A single- or double-headed needle is used to transfer dissolved medication in a vial to an I.V. bottle with intact vacuum. A syringe with a filter needle or filter straw can be used to transfer medication in an ampul to a bottle or bag; an ampul transfer device can be used to add medication only to a bottle with intact vacuum.

Before adding any drug to an I.V. solution, make sure to establish compatibility of the solution with the drug. Avoid adding drugs to blood—this complicates identifying the source of an adverse reaction.

Follow these guidelines when adding drugs to an I.V. solution:
• Check hospital policy to see if you're allowed to add the drug to the I.V. solution. If so, find out how the drug to be added is packaged, and then obtain the appropriate transfer device and any necessary diluent. Check the compatibility and dosage of the drug, diluent, and I.V. solution.

• When you remove the metal cap from an I.V. bottle, you'll see a protective rubber disk. This disk is sterile and needn't be swabbed with alcohol for its first puncture. Drugs can be injected through it with a needle. When you're ready to connect the I.V. tubing, remove the disk to expose the sterile bottle diaphragm. You should hear a pop when you remove the disk (unless you've already punctured it), assuring the container's sterility. The sterile bottle top needn't be swabbed first.

To use a syringe and needle:
• Remove the protective metal cap from the drug vial. You don't have to wipe the vial top with alcohol before the first puncture, since it's sterile. After the first puncture, however, wipe the top with a sterile alcohol sponge before each subsequent puncture.
• If the drug to be added is a powder, aspirate the correct amount of diluent into the syringe and inject it into the drug vial. Roll the vial between your hands to dissolve all particles.
• If the I.V. container is a bottle, remove the protective metal cap, leaving the rubber seal intact. If the I.V. container is a bag, swab

Continuous Drip Method
Continued

the rubber-stoppered port.
• Inject the drug and gently rotate the bottle or squeeze the bag to mix the solution.
To use a single-headed needle or pin:
• Remove the protective cap from the needle or pin on top of the drug vial. Then remove the metal cap from the I.V. bottle.
• Invert the medication vial and insert the pin into the I.V. bottle's main port so the vacuum draws the drug into the bottle. Remove the vial and gently rotate the bottle to mix the solution.
To use a double-headed needle or pin:
• Remove the protective cap from the drug vial and swab the rubber seal with an alcohol sponge, if desired.
• If the drug to be added is a powder, add the appropriate diluent with a needle and syringe and roll the vial between your hands to dissolve all particles.
• Remove the outside cover of the double-headed needle to expose the shorter needle. Insert this needle into the drug vial and remove the second half of the needle cover, exposing the longer needle.

• If you're adding medication to an I.V. bottle, remove the protective metal cap. (If you're using an I.V. bag, wipe the rubber-stoppered port with an alcohol sponge.) Invert the medication vial, and insert the longer needle into the center hole of the appropriate seal. The vacuum then draws the drug into the I.V. container. Remove the vial and gently rotate the container to mix the solution.
To use a syringe with a filter needle or straw:
• If the I.V. container is a bottle, remove the protective metal cap and wipe the seal or port with alcohol, if desired.
• Place the filter needle or straw on the syringe. Then wipe the ampul neck with an alcohol sponge, wrap it in a gauze pad, and snap off the neck, directing the force away from your body.
• Aspirate the ampul contents with the syringe. Then replace the filter needle or straw with a 25G 1″ needle.
• Inject the drug into the I.V. container and rotate the container to mix the solution.

Continued

PARENTERAL MEDICATIONS

Continuous Drip Method
Continued

To use an ampul transfer device:
• Remove the protective metal cap from the I.V. bottle and wipe the rubber seal with an alcohol sponge, if desired.
• Swab the ampul neck with alcohol, wrap it in a gauze pad, and snap it off, directing the force away from your body.
• Attach a 25G 1″ needle to the adapter end of the transfer device. Completely insert the opposite end of the device into the ampul.
• Insert the needle into the injection site on the I.V. bottle's rubber seal. The vacuum draws the drug into the bottle.
• Tilt the ampul to keep the tip of the device covered with the drug. Then rotate the bottle to mix the solution.

After preparing the solution:
• Recheck the drug dose and I.V. solution to prevent error.
• Connect the I.V. administration set or sterile protective cap (provided by the manufacturer) to the I.V. container to prevent contamination.
• Fill out the medication-added label and place it on the I.V. container. The label should include the date, drug dose, infusion rate, your initials, and the time the drug was added to the I.V. container.

Special considerations
• Maintain sterile technique throughout this procedure.
• Since the vacuum of an I.V. bottle remains intact for only one puncture, use a syringe and needle to transfer any other drugs to the bottle.
• When making multiple drug transfers, add only one drug at a time. Always add the most concentrated drug first and any colored drugs last. Mix the solution thoroughly and examine it after adding each drug for precipitation, discoloration, or cloudiness.
• To add a drug to an I.V. solution that has already been hung, always close the flow clamp to prevent delivering a bolus of the drug to the patient. Insert a syringe and needle into the injection site of a vented I.V. bottle or the injection port of an I.V. bag after wiping it with alcohol. Always rotate the container gently to mix the solution. Then open the flow clamp and adjust the flow rate.

PARENTERAL MEDICATIONS

Infusing Medications Through a Secondary I.V. Line

A secondary I.V. line is a complete I.V. set—container, tubing, and needle—connected to the injection port of a primary line instead of to the I.V. catheter or needle. It can be used for continuous or intermittent drug infusion. When used continuously, a secondary I.V. line permits drug infusion and titration while the primary line maintains a constant total infusion rate. When used intermittently, it's commonly called a piggyback set; in this case, the primary line maintains venous access between drug doses. Antibiotics are most commonly administered by intermittent (piggyback) infusion.

I.V. pumps may be used to maintain constant infusion rates, especially with a drug such as lidocaine. A pump allows more accurate titration of drug dosage and helps maintain venous access, because the drug is delivered under sufficient pressure to prevent clot formation in the I.V. cannula.

A secondary I.V. line shouldn't be connected to a hyperalimentation line, be-cause of the risk of contamination.

Follow these guidelines when using a secondary I.V. line:
• Check drug compatibility with the primary solution. See if the primary line has a secondary injection port. If it doesn't, and the medications will be given regularly, replace the I.V. set with a new one that has a secondary injection port.
• If necessary, add the drug to the secondary I.V. solution. To do so, remove any seals from the secondary container and wipe the main port with a sterile alcohol sponge. Inject the prescribed medication and gently agitate the solution to mix the medication thoroughly. Properly label the I.V. mixture. Insert the administration set spike and attach the needle. Remove the needle cover, open the flow clamp, and prime the line. Then close the flow clamp and replace the needle cover.
• If the drug is incompatible with the primary I.V. solution,

Continued

Infusing Medications Through a Secondary I.V. Line
Continued

replace the solution with normal saline and flush the line before starting the drug infusion. Many hospital protocols require removing the primary (incompatible) I.V. solution and inserting a sterile I.V. plug into the container until you're ready to rehang it. This will maintain the solution's sterility and prevent someone else from inadvertently restarting the incompatible solution before the line is flushed with normal saline solution.

• Hang the secondary container and wipe the injection port of the primary line with an alcohol sponge.

• Insert the needle from the secondary line into the injection port and tape it securely to the primary line.

• To run the secondary container solely, lower the primary container with an extension hook. To run both containers simultaneously, place them at the same height.

• Open the clamp and adjust the drip rate. For *continuous infusion,* set the secondary solution to the desired drip rate; then adjust the primary solution to achieve the desired total infusion rate.

• For *intermittent infusion,* adjust the primary drip rate as required upon completion of the secondary solution. If the secondary solution tubing is being reused, close the clamp on the tubing and follow the institution's policy: either remove the needle and replace it with a new one, or leave it securely taped in the injection port and label it with the time it was first used. In this case, also leave the empty container in place until you replace it with a new medication dose at the prescribed time. If the tubing won't be reused, discard it appropriately with the I.V. container.

Special considerations
• Repeated punctures of the secondary injection port can cause an imperfect seal, with possible leakage or contamination.

Continued

Infusing Medications Through a Secondary I.V. Line
Continued

A piggyback set—used solely for intermittent drug infusion—includes a small I.V. bottle, short tubing, and usually a macrodrip system. It connects into a primary line's upper Y port (piggyback port). For the set to work, you must use an extension hook to position the primary I.V. container below the piggyback container, as shown.

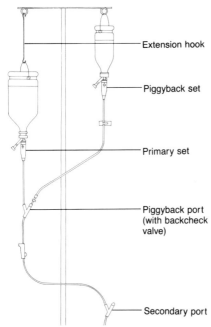

Extension hook

Piggyback set

Primary set

Piggyback port (with backcheck valve)

Secondary port

Using an Intermittent Infusion Injection Device

An intermittent infusion injection device—or heparin lock—eliminates the need for multiple venipunctures or to maintain venous access with a continuous I.V. infusion. It allows intermittent administration through this device by infusion or by the I.V. bolus or I.V. push injection methods. Dilute heparin solution may be injected as the final step in this procedure to prevent clotting in the device. When this is done, the device must be flushed with normal saline solution before and after the prescribed medication is administered in case the heparin and the medication are incompatible. The device may then be reflushed with the heparin solution.

Keep these important considerations in mind when using the device:
• Stop the injection immediately if you feel any resistance, which indicates that the device is occluded. If this occurs, insert a new intermittent infusion device.
• If you're giving a bolus injection of a drug that's incompatible with saline, such as diazepam, flush the device with bacteriostatic water.
• In some institutions, the device is flushed with 2 to 3 ml of normal saline solution instead of heparin flush solution to prevent clotting in the cannula.

Intermittent infusion devices should be changed regularly, according to hospital policy (usually every 48 to 72 hours).

Male adapter plugs allow conversion of an existing I.V. line to an intermittent infusion set. To do this, prime the male adapter plug with dilute heparin. Then, clamp the I.V. tubing, remove the administration set from the catheter or needle hub, and insert the male adapter plug. Next, inject the remaining dilute heparin to fill the line and to prevent clot formation.

Detecting I.V. Solution Incompatibility

To avoid I.V. solution incompatibility, administer medications separately whenever possible. To minimize incompatibilities, use a heparin lock to infuse multiple doses of a drug that's incompatible with other parenteral drugs.

If several incompatible drugs must be infused through the same I.V. line, clear the tubing between doses with a solution compatible with each drug.

When medications must be administered concurrently or mixed in the same large-volume parenteral solution, refer to the following guidelines:
• When preparing a drug, follow manufacturer's instructions meticulously because the preservatives used in some diluents may be incompatible with the drug.
• When reconstituting I.V. drugs and inspecting for a precipitate, don't shake the container; rotate or swirl it instead. This action prevents air-bubble entrapment and foaming, which impair accurate drug-dose measurement in syringes and trigger air exclusion alarms when solutions are administered by infusion pump. Also, air bubbles may be mistaken for particles in the solution.
• When reconstituting a drug, thoroughly mix it before administering or adding it to a solution.
• When mixing drugs in a large-volume parenteral solution, add one

drug at a time; then mix and examine the solution before adding other drugs. Thorough mixing before adding other drugs prevents layering. Also, avoid adding more than two drugs whenever possible.
• Chemical reactions depend on concentration. Minimize these reactions by adding the most concentrated or most soluble drug to the large-volume parenteral solution first.
• Some precipitates are too fine or too clear to be detected, or are the same color as the solution. When you swirl or rotate the container, inspect for a precipitate in good light against both a dark and light background.
• Watch for color changes in the membrane of any I.V. filter device, indicating drug incompatibility not visible in the solution. This reaction becomes visible as the drug is trapped and accumulates in the filter chamber.
• If you detect a physical change, such as a precipitate or discoloration, don't administer the admixture. Notify the pharmacist.
• Avoid administering intermittent medications along with IVH (intravenous hyperalimentation) solutions through a central venous catheter. Doing so risks contamination and incompatibilities. Use a secondary line for these drugs.
• Don't mix additives with blood or blood products.

PARENTERAL MEDICATIONS

Managing I.V. Extravasation

PARENTERAL MEDICATIONS

Extravasation, leakage of infused solution from a vein into surrounding tissue, results from a needle puncture of a vascular wall or leakage around a venipuncture site. Extravasation causes local pain and itching, edema, blanching, and decreased skin temperature in the affected extremity. Extravasation of intravenous solution may be referred to as infiltration, because the fluid infiltrates the tissues. Extravasation of a small amount of isotonic fluid or a nonirritating drug usually causes only minor discomfort. However, extravasation of some drugs can severely damage tissue through irritative, sclerotic, vesicant, corrosive, or vasoconstrictive action. In these cases, immediate measures must be taken to minimize tissue damage, preventing the need for skin grafts or, rarely, possible amputation.

Treatment of extravasation of I.V. solutions and nonirritating drugs involves routine comfort measures, such as application of warm soaks. Treatment of extravasation of corrosive drugs requires emergency treatment to prevent severe tissue necrosis. However, the following guidelines may be used.

Treatment of extravasation is controversial, so check your hospital protocol before proceeding. Follow these guidelines when managing I.V. extravasation:

● Stop the infusion immediately, but *don't* remove the I.V. needle. Carefully estimate the amount of extravasated solution, and notify the doctor.

● Disconnect the tubing from the I.V. needle. Attach a 5-ml syringe to the needle and try to withdraw 3 to 5 ml of blood to remove any medication or blood in the tubing or needle and provide a path to the infiltrated tissues.

● Cleanse the area around the extravasation site with an alcohol sponge or gauze sponge soaked in antiseptic solution. Then, insert the needle of an empty tuberculin syringe into the subcutaneous tissue around the site and gently aspirate

Continued

Managing I.V. Extravasation
Continued

as much of the solution as possible from the tissue.
• As indicated and if ordered, instill the antidote into the same area. Then, if ordered, slowly instill an anti-inflammatory drug subcutaneously to help reduce inflammation and edema.
• Remove the I.V. needle.
• Apply cold compresses to the affected area for 24 hours, or apply an ice pack for 20 minutes every 4 hours to cause vasoconstriction that may localize the drug and slow cell metabolism. After 24 hours, apply warm compresses and elevate the affected extremity to reduce discomfort and promote fluid reabsorption. If the extravasated drug is a vasoconstrictor, such as norepinephrine or metaraminol bitartrate, apply warm compresses only.
• Continuously monitor the I.V. site for signs of abscess or necrosis.

Special considerations
Know the antidote (if any) for an I.V. drug that can cause tissue necrosis if extravasation occurs. Make sure you're familiar with your institution's policy regarding the administration of such drugs and their antidotes.

Tell the patient to report any discomfort at the I.V. site. During infusion, frequently check the I.V. site for signs of infiltration.

Drugs Hazardous on Extravasation

The following drugs are commonly associated with tissue necrosis when they extravasate:
amphotericin B (Fungizone)
daunorubicin (Cerubidine)
dopamine (Intropin)
doxorubicin (Adriamycin)
mechlorethamine, nitrogen mustard (Mustargen)
metaraminol bitartrate (Aramine)
mithramycin (Mithracin)
mitomycin (Mutamycin)
nitroprusside sodium (Nipride)
norepinephrine (Levophed)
potassium chloride
vancomycin (Vancocin)
vinblastine (Velban)
vincristine (Oncovin)

Other Venous Access Devices

Although a standard I.V. line's most commonly used to administer I.V. medications, other devices may be used in special circumstances. Read what follows to review these devices.

Indwelling catheter

Such devices as the Hickman or Broviac catheter maintain venous access for drawing blood and administering I.V. hyperalimentation (IVH) or medication. A surgeon inserts the catheter while the patient's under local anesthesia. Usually, the catheter's proximal end rests in the right atrium, while its distal end passes through the superior vena cava, the cephalic vein, and a subcutaneous tunnel before exiting the body between the clavicle and the nipple. (Alternatively, the catheter can be introduced into a femoral vein and fed into the inferior vena cava to the right atrium. The catheter tunnel then lies at the abdomen rather than the chest.)

An indwelling catheter requires irrigation with heparin between infusions and special dressing changes to prevent infection. Although this catheter's not permanent, it does provide long-term venous access.

Central venous catheter

This device maintains venous access for drawing blood and administering IVH, medications, blood, or fluids. The doctor inserts the catheter through the subclavian vein (or, less commonly, the jugular vein) into the superior vena cava. Once in place, the central venous line also allows vena cava blood pressure monitoring. In many cases, a central venous catheter port's also contained in a pulmonary artery catheter.

Although most central venous catheters have just one lumen, the quad-lumen I.V. catheter has four. The four lumens allow you to administer several drugs at once. And because the catheter's inserted into a large vein, blood's volume and natural turbulence mix the solutions and dilute them quickly. That means you can avoid problems caused by incompatible infusions. Also, instead of caring for multiple I.V. sites, you care for only one.

The lumens, which run the catheter's length, differ in diameter and color. To infuse highly viscous fluids, such as blood or albumin, you'd use the two wide lumens—color-coded blue and yellow. For normal I.V. solutions, you'd use the two narrow lumens—red and white.

Continued

Other Venous Access Devices
Continued

Implanted infusion port

For a patient who's at risk for, or who has, damaged veins, this device can provide venous access for drawing blood and administering medication or IVH. Usually, a surgeon implants the port and its Silastic catheter, which he tunnels to a central vein. The port itself fits in a subcutaneous pocket over a bony prominence, such as the distal third of the clavicle.

Because the infusion port's implanted under the skin, it reduces the infection risk and minimizes body image changes. It can last indefinitely, requires intermittent irrigation with heparin, and never needs a dressing. However, it's harder to manipulate than the indwelling catheter and requires the patient to insert a needle through his skin to administer drugs or fluid.

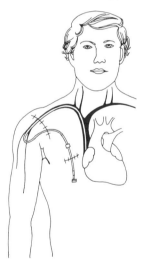

Indwelling catheter

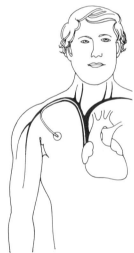

Implanted infusion port

Intraarterial Infusion

Intraarterial infusion can deliver an antineoplastic drug through a catheter in a major artery directly into a localized, inoperable tumor. This procedure allows a high drug concentration to reach the tumor with little dilution by the circulatory system and before metabolic breakdown by the liver or kidneys. The intraarterial catheter is directly implanted surgically or threaded through a peripheral artery into branches of the celiac artery for liver tumors, into the external carotid artery for head and neck tumors, and into the internal carotid artery for brain tumors.

Intraarterial infusion can also deliver vasopressin to the site of GI bleeding. Usually, the catheter is threaded from a peripheral site to the left gastric, celiac, or mesenteric artery, depending on the bleeding site.

To prevent blood backflow and clotting, infusion of heparinized saline begins after direct implantation of the catheter in the operating room or after insertion and confirmation of placement in the X-ray department. Equipment for initial infusion must accompany the patient to either location. To allow assessment of response, intraarterial infusion generally begins after the patient returns to the patient care unit.

To monitor the patient after catheter insertion:

• If applicable, check the level of the pressure cuff. It should read at least 150 mm Hg and must be higher than the patient's systolic blood pressure (but not over 300 mm Hg) to ensure an adequate drip rate for the infused solution. After checking the pressure, close the inflation flow valve to prevent air leaks from the pressure cuff. If leaks do occur, clamp the tubing between the pressure cuff and the bulb with a hemostat. (To protect the rubber tubing from damage, wrap a 4″ × 4″ gauze sponge around the tubing before attaching the hemostat.)

• Monitor the site for bleeding, ecchymosis, hematoma,

Continued

Intraarterial Infusion
Continued

or catheter movement. Infection can follow catheter insertion, but generally appears several days later.
• Watch for changes in catheter length.

To change a bag with an infusion pump:
• Stop the infusion, turn the stopcock off, remove the tubing spike from the old bag, and insert it into the new one after cleansing the port with a sterile alcohol sponge.
• Hang the new bag, turn the stopcock on, and start the infusion pump.

To change a bag with a pressure cuff:
• Close the flow clamp, turn the stopcock off, and turn the pressure-release valve counterclockwise to deflate the pressure cuff.
• Remove the old bag from the pressure cuff and the tubing spike from the old bag. Put in the new bag, and slip the tab through the hole on the top of the bag.

• Wipe the port with an alcohol sponge. Insert the tubing spike and hang the new equipment on the I.V. pole.
• Turn the pressure-release valve clockwise to prevent air from escaping and inflate the pressure cuff as necessary—to 150 to 300 mm Hg—to ensure an adequate drip rate.
• Open the stopcock and the flow clamp, and adjust to the desired drip rate.

Special considerations
• When possible, change the tubing every 24 hours with the solution.
• Change the dressing every 24 hours or when wet, following hospital policy.
• Observe the infusion site for catheter displacement, edema, bleeding, ecchymosis, hematoma, and infection.
• Thrombus formation, the most common complication of intraarterial infusion, usually requires catheter removal by the doctor.

PARENTERAL MEDICATIONS

Injecting Intrathecal Medications

An intrathecal injection allows direct administration of medication into the subarachnoid space of the spinal canal. Certain drugs—such as anti-infectives, or anti-neoplastics used to treat meningeal leukemia—are administered by this route because they can't readily penetrate the subdural membrane through the bloodstream. Intrathecal injection may also be used to deliver anesthetics such as lidocaine hydrochloride to achieve regional anesthesia as in spinal anesthesia or epidural block.

An invasive procedure performed by a doctor under sterile conditions, with the nurse assisting, intrathecal injection requires informed patient consent. The injection site is usually between the third and fourth (or fourth and fifth) lumbar vertebrae.

Follow these guidelines when administering intrathecal medications:
• Make sure the patient or a responsible family member has signed the consent form.
• Reinforce the doctor's explanation of the procedure to the patient. Tell him that he may experience a stinging sensation when the anesthetic is injected.
• Tell the patient to void just before the procedure because he may have to stay in bed several hours afterward.

• Place the patient in the right or left lateral position, as directed by the doctor. Use pillows, if permissible, to make him comfortable. Be sure the puncture site is exposed.
• After the doctor anesthetizes the skin and subcutaneous tissue, he inserts a lumbar puncture needle into the lumbar space. At this point, he may collect some spinal fluid for laboratory analysis.
• The doctor attaches the syringe containing the prescribed medication to the lumbar puncture needle and injects the medication into the subarachnoid space.
• After the needle is withdrawn, apply an adhesive bandage to the site.
• Press gently on the injection site for a couple of minutes, as directed, to prevent medication seepage.
• Place the patient in the position ordered by the doctor.

Special considerations
• If the patient can't maintain the correct position, help him maintain back flexion by gently but firmly grasping him behind the neck and knees.
• Encourage the patient to drink fluids, as permitted, to help replace any spinal fluid loss.
• An infusion port, the Ommaya reservoir, may be implanted beneath the patient's scalp to administer long-term intrathecal drugs, such as chemotherapy.

New Drug Delivery Systems

Thanks to recent break-throughs in drug delivery technology, drugs can now be delivered by systems other than the traditional ones. Read what follows to find out about these new drug delivery systems.

Externally applied drug delivery

This category now includes elastomeric infusors and ophthalmic wafers. The *elastomeric infusor* is a disposable I.V. pump now used mainly to deliver cancer chemotherapy. Worn on the abdomen, the device frees the patient from attachment to a pole-mounted I.V. bottle. *Ocusert,* which helps treat patients with glaucoma, is a thin, flexible wafer placed under the eyelid. It delivers a weekly dose of pilocarpine, a powerful miotic drug.

Oral drug delivery

The *OROS* (oral osmotic) system consists of a solid drug core coated with a semipermeable polymer membrane that contains a single tiny orifice. After it's swallowed, the system functions as a minute osmotic pump, admitting water through the membrane and releasing medication through the orifice at a controlled rate for up to 24 hours.

The *Pennkinetic* drug delivery system, now used for several liquid cough and cold medicines, employs the principle of ion exchange to control drug release. Drug molecules and an ion-exchange polymer are bound together to form a drug-polymer complex. This complex is coated with a semipermeable membrane of varying thickness, depending on the drug-release rate. Sodium and potassium ions in body fluids penetrate the membrane and displace the drug molecules on the surface of the drug-polymer complex, releasing the drug at a controlled rate.

Implantable drug delivery

These systems also hold great promise. For example, an intrauterine contraceptive device called *Progestasert* releases controlled progesterone amounts directly into the uterus.

Choosing the Venipuncture Site

In most cases, the best sites for venipuncture on a patient are (in order of preference) his lower arm and hand, his upper arm, and his antecubital fossa. Avoid performing venipuncture in the patient's legs, because he'll run a greater risk of developing thrombophlebitis and an embolism. Whenever possible, use the distal end of the vein. But first, ask yourself these questions:

• *How long will I.V. therapy last?* For short-term therapy, use the patient's left arm or hand if he's right-handed, his right arm or hand if he's left-handed. For long-term therapy, alternate the patient's arms and avoid sites over joints. (If your patient will be receiving long-term I.V. therapy, get maximum use from his arm veins by starting the therapy in a hand vein, then switching to sites farther up his arm, as necessary.)

• *What kind of I.V. solution's been ordered?* For highly acidic, alkaline, or hypertonic infusions, use a large vein to adequately dilute the infusion. A small peripheral vein may become irritated. Rapid infusions also require larger veins.

• *What size needle or cannula*

are you using? If the solution's highly viscous, you'll need a large-bore needle or cannula. Then, choose a vein that's big enough to accommodate it.

• *Is the vein full, soft, and unobstructed?* Palpate the patient's veins to find one that's not crooked, hardened, scarred, or inflamed. If you must perform venipuncture in the patient's leg, avoid using a varicose vein. However, if you *must* use one, elevate the patient's leg during the infusion.

• *Does your patient have any specific problems or injuries that require special consideration?* Avoid veins in irritated, infected, or injured areas. The added stress of venipuncture may cause complications.

• *How old is the patient?* If your patient's an adolescent or an adult, his hand or lower arm will probably provide the best site. But if you're giving I.V. therapy to an infant, insert the needle in a scalp vein, where it can be protected. Then, cover the site with an inverted paper cup that's been slotted on one side to accommodate the tube. Tape the cup to the infant's head with nonallergenic tape.

Continued

Choosing the Venipuncture Site
Continued

Antecubital fossa—Left arm

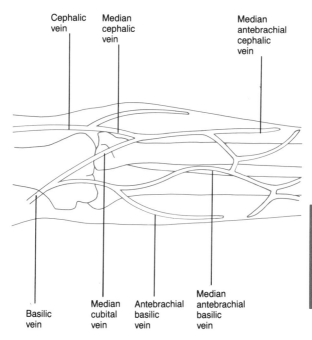

I.V. THERAPY

Preparing for I.V. Therapy

Before initiating I.V. therapy, make sure to properly select and assemble the equipment to ensure accurate delivery of the I.V. solution. Selection of an I.V. administration set reflects the rate and type of infusion and the type of I.V. solution container. Two types of drip system are available: the macrodrip and the microdrip set. The macrodrip set can deliver a solution in large quantities and at rapid rates because it delivers a larger amount of solution with each drop than the microdrip set. The microdrip set delivers a smaller quantity of solution with each drop. Administration tubing with a secondary injection port permits separate or simultaneous infusion of two solutions; tubing with a piggyback port and a back-check valve permits intermittent infusion of a secondary solution and, on its completion, automatic return to infusion of the primary solution. Use vented I.V. tubing for a solution contained in a non-vented bottle; nonvented tubing, for a solution contained in a bag or vented bottle.

Follow these guidelines when preparing for I.V. therapy:
• Verify the type, volume, and expiration date of the I.V. solution. Discard any outdated solution. If the solution's contained in a glass bottle, inspect for chips or cracks; if it's in a plastic bag, squeeze to detect leaks. Examine the I.V. solution for particles, abnormal discoloration, and cloudiness. If present, discard the solution and notify the pharmacy or dispensing department. If ordered, add medication to the solution, and place a completed medication-added label on the container. Remove the administration set from its box and observe for cracks, holes, and missing clamps.
• Slide the flow clamp of the administration set close to the drip chamber or injection port, and close the clamp.
To prepare a nonvented bottle:
• Remove the bottle's metal cap and inner disk, if present.
• Place the bottle on a stable surface, and wipe the rubber stopper with an alcohol sponge.
• Remove the protective cap from the administration set spike, and push the spike through the center of the bottle's rubber stopper. Avoid twisting or angling the spike to prevent pieces of the stopper from breaking off and falling into the solution.
• Invert the bottle. If its vacuum is intact, you'll hear a hissing sound and see air bubbles rise (this may not occur if you've already added medication). If it's not intact, discard the bottle.

Continued

Preparing for I.V. Therapy
Continued

• Hang the bottle on the I.V. pole, and squeeze the drip chamber until it is half full.

To prepare a vented bottle:

• Remove the bottle's metal cap and latex diaphragm to release the vacuum. If the vacuum isn't intact (except after medication has been added), discard the bottle.

• Place the bottle on a stable surface, and wipe the rubber stopper with an alcohol sponge.

• Remove the protective cap from the administration set spike, and push the spike through the insertion port next to the air vent tube opening.

• Hang the bottle on the I.V. pole, and squeeze the drip chamber until it's half full.

To prepare a bag:

• Place the bag on a flat, stable surface or hang it on an I.V. pole. Then, remove the protective cap or tear tab from the tubing insertion port, and wipe the port with an alcohol sponge.

• Remove the protective cap from the administration set spike.

• Holding the port carefully and firmly with one hand, quickly insert the spike with your other hand.

• Hang the bag, if not already done, and squeeze the drip chamber until it's half full.

To prime the I.V. tubing and conclude preparation:

• If desired, attach a filter to the opposite end of the I.V. tubing, and follow the manufacturer's instructions for filling and priming.

• If you're not using a filter, remove the protective cap on the tubing. Then, while maintaining the sterility of the end of the tubing, hold it over a wastebasket or sink, and open the flow clamp.

• Leave the clamp open until I.V. solution flows through the entire length of tubing, forcing out all air. Invert all Y-injection sites and backcheck valves, and tap them, if necessary, to fill them with solution.

• After priming the tubing, close the clamp and replace the protective cover. Then, loop the tubing over the I.V. pole.

• Label the container with the patient's name and room number, the date and time, the container number, the ordered duration of infusion, and your initials.

Special considerations

• Always use aseptic technique when preparing I.V. components. If you contaminate the administration set or container, replace it with a new one to prevent introducing contaminants into the system.

• If necessary, you can use vented tubing with a vented bottle. To do this, don't remove the latex diaphragm. Instead, insert the spike into the larger indentation in the diaphragm.

I.V. THERAPY

Guidelines for Using In-Line I.V. Filters

An in-line I.V. filter, such as the 0.22-micron model, removes pathogens and particles from I.V. solutions, helping to reduce the risk of infusion phlebitis. Because a filter is expensive and its installation in an I.V. line is cumbersome and time-consuming, it's not routinely used. Consequently, many institutions require use of a filter only when an admixture is being administered. However, if you're unsure whether or not to use a filter, follow these guidelines.

Use in-line I.V. filters:
- for any infusion to an immunodeficient patient
- for hyperalimentation
- when using additives comprising many separate particles, such as antibiotics requiring reconstitution, or when administering several additives

- when using rubber injection sites or plastic diaphragms frequently
- when phlebitis is likely to occur.

Be sure to change in-line I.V. filters at least every 24 hours. If you don't, bacteria trapped in the filter release endotoxin, a pyrogen small enough to pass through the filter into the bloodstream.

Avoid using in-line I.V. filters:
- when administering solutions with large particles that will clog the filter and stop I.V. flow; for example, blood and its components, suspensions (such as amphotericin B), fat emulsions (such as Liposyn), and high–molecular-volume plasma expanders (such as Dextran)
- when administering a small dosage of a drug because the filter may absorb it.

Needles and Catheters for Peripheral Lines

Winged infusion set
Purpose: short-term therapy for any cooperative adult patient; therapy of any duration for an infant or child or for an elderly patient with fragile or sclerotic veins
Advantages: lower incidence of infection and phlebitis than with catheters; easy to insert and secure
Disadvantage: risk of irritation or puncture of vein from movement

Inside-the-needle catheter
Purpose: long-term therapy for the active or agitated patient; also used for central venous insertion
Advantages: puncture of vein less likely than with a needle; more comfortable for the patient once it's in place; available in many lengths; most plastic catheters contain radiopaque thread, permitting easy location

Continued

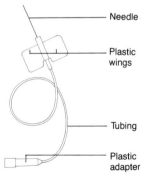

— Needle

— Plastic wings

— Tubing

— Plastic adapter

Winged infusion set

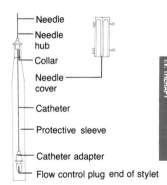

— Needle
— Needle hub
— Collar
— Needle cover
— Catheter
— Protective sleeve
— Catheter adapter
— Flow control plug end of stylet

Inside-the-needle catheter

I.V. THERAPY

Needles and Catheters for Peripheral Lines
Continued

Disadvantages: greater incidence of infection and phlebitis than with a needle or shorter over-the-needle catheter; some hospitals may not allow nurses to insert it; catheter easily severed; kinking possible due to joint flexion

Over-the-needle catheter

Purpose: long-term therapy for the active or agitated patient

Advantages: puncture of vein less likely than with a needle; more comfortable for the patient once it's in place; contains radiopaque thread for easy location; easy to insert

Disadvantages: greater incidence of infection and phlebitis than with a needle; kinking possible due to joint flexion.

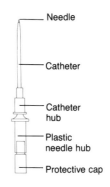

Over-the-needle catheter

Inserting a Peripheral I.V. Line

One of the most commonly performed procedures, insertion of a peripheral I.V. line involves selection of a cannula and insertion site, application of a tourniquet, preparation of the site, and venipuncture. Selection of a cannula and site depends on the type of solution; the frequency and duration of infusion; the patient's age, size, and condition; and the patency and location of available veins. The most favorable venipuncture sites are the cephalic, basilic, and antebrachial veins in the lower arm and the veins in the hand's dorsal surface; the least favorable are the leg and foot veins because of the increased thrombophlebitis risk.

Use of a peripheral line allows administration of fluids, medication, blood, and blood components and maintenance of an open vein. Insertion at a particular site is contraindicated in a sclerotic vein and in the presence of burns or an arteriovenous fistula.

Follow these steps when inserting a peripheral I.V. line:

• Wash your hands thoroughly to prevent infection. Then, explain the procedure to the patient to ensure cooperation and reduce anxiety, which can cause a vasomotor response resulting in venous constriction.
• Select the puncture site— preferably a vein in the nondominant arm, but never one in an edematous or impaired arm or leg. For fluid replacement, choose a small vein unless a large vein will be needed for subsequent therapy; this leaves the large veins available for emergency infusion. If long-term therapy is anticipated, start with a vein at the most distal site so you can move upward as needed for further I.V. insertion sites. For infusion of a caustic medication, choose a site away from joints, with plenty of subcutaneous tissue. Be sure the vein can accommodate the cannula if used.
• Wrap a tourniquet 4″ to 8″ (10 to 20 cm) above the intended puncture site to dilate the vein.
• Lightly palpate the vein with

Continued

I.V. THERAPY

Inserting a Peripheral I.V. Line
Continued

your index and middle fingers.
• If the vein is easily palpable but not sufficiently dilated, one or more of the following techniques may help raise the vein: Tap gently with your finger over the vein, place the extremity in a dependent position for several seconds, or, if you have selected a vein in the arm or hand, tell the patient to open and close his fist several times.
• Cleanse the venipuncture site.
• Grasp the needle or catheter. If you're using a *winged infusion set,* hold the short edges of the wings, with the bevel facing upward, between the thumb and forefinger of your dominant hand. Then, squeeze the wings together.

If you're using an *over-the-needle catheter,* grasp the plastic hub with your dominant hand, remove the cover, and examine the catheter tip. If the edge isn't smooth, discard and replace the device.

If you're using an *inside-the-needle catheter,* grasp the needle hub with one hand, and unsnap the needle cover. Then, rotate the catheter device until the bevel faces upward.

To insert the needle or catheter using the indirect method, follow these steps:
• Using the thumb of your opposite hand, stretch the skin taut below the puncture site to stabilize the vein.
• Hold the needle at a 45° angle slightly below and to one side of the puncture site, with the needle pointing in the direction of venous flow.
• Push the needle through the skin until you meet resistance, but avoid penetrating the vein. Now, lower the needle to a 15° to 20° angle (almost level with the skin's surface) and slowly pierce the vein; you should feel it pop.

(*Note:* You can also use the direct insertion method by inserting the needle or catheter into the vein in one quick motion.)
• When you observe blood backflow behind the needle, tilt the needle slightly upward and advance it farther into the vein to prevent puncture of the posterior vein wall.
• If you're using a *winged*

Continued

Inserting a Peripheral I.V. Line
Continued

infusion set, advance the needle fully, if possible, and hold it in place. Attach the administration set, then open the clamp slightly, and check for free flow. Then, tape the winged infusion set and tubing in place according to hospital policy.

If you're using an *over-the-needle catheter,* pull back on the needle with one hand and advance the catheter fully with your opposite hand. Then, apply pressure to the vein beyond the catheter tip to prevent blood leakage, and remove the needle. Release the tourniquet, and attach the administration set to the catheter hub. Then, open the administration set clamp slightly, and check for free flow. Tape the catheter according to hospital policy.

If you're using an *inside-the-needle catheter,* remove the tourniquet, hold the needle in place with one hand, and, with your opposite hand, grasp the catheter through the protective sleeve. Then, slowly thread the catheter through the needle until the hub is within the needle col-

lar. Then, withdraw the metal needle, and cover it with the protector. Remove the stylet and protective sleeve, and attach the administration set to the catheter hub. Open the administration set clamp slightly, and check for free flow. Then tape the catheter according to hospital policy.

● Apply the I.V. site dressing as specified by hospital policy.

● Loop the I.V. tubing on the extremity, and secure the tubing with tape. The loop allows some slack to prevent dislodgement of the catheter from tension on the line.

● Label the last piece of tape with the type and gauge of needle or catheter, the date and time of insertion, and your initials. Adjust the flow rate, as ordered.

Special considerations
● If you fail to see blood backflow after entering the vein, pull back slightly and rotate the cannula. If you still fail to see backflow, remove the cannula and try again. If you still don't succeed, ask another nurse to perform the venipuncture.

I.V. THERAPY

Managing I.V. Therapy Complications

INFILTRATION

Possible causes
• Needle or catheter displacement
• Puncture of the vein
Signs and symptoms
• Cool skin, swelling, and discomfort around site
• Edema of entire arm or leg
• Absence of blood flashback
• Sluggish flow rate
Intervention
• Discontinue the infusion, and remove the catheter immediately.
• If infiltration is detected within 30 minutes of onset and swelling is slight, apply ice. Otherwise, apply warm, wet compresses to promote absorption, and elevate the affected arm or leg.

PHLEBITIS

Possible causes
• Injury to vein
• Irritation to vein
Signs and symptoms
• Edema along the course of the affected vein

• Sore, hard, cordlike, and warm vein; possibly a red line above the venipuncture site
Intervention
• Discontinue the infusion, and remove the needle or catheter immediately.
• Apply warm, moist compresses.
• Notify the doctor.

CIRCULATORY OVERLOAD

Possible causes
• Excessive or too rapid administration
Signs and symptoms
• Increased blood pressure and central venous pressure
• Venous dilatation, especially of neck veins
• Rapid breathing, shortness of breath
Intervention
• Slow the infusion to a keep-vein-open rate.
• Raise the patient's head, and keep him warm.
• Monitor vital signs.
• Notify the doctor.

Continued

Managing I.V. Therapy Complications
Continued

AIR EMBOLISM

Possible causes
• Empty solution container
• Air in tubing
• Loose connections, allowing air to enter tubing
Signs and symptoms
• Decreased blood pressure
• Weak, rapid pulse
• Cyanosis
• Loss of consciousness
Intervention
• Turn the patient to the left side so any small air bubbles entering the heart can be absorbed in the pulmonary artery.
• Notify the doctor immediately.
• Check the system for leaks.

CATHETER EMBOLISM
(most common with inside-the-needle catheters)

Possible causes
• Removal of the catheter before the needle
• Attempting to rethread the catheter with a needle
• Unsecured catheter
Signs and symptoms
• Discomfort along the vein
• Cyanosis
• Decreased blood pressure
• Weak, rapid pulse
• Loss of consciousness
Intervention
• Discontinue the infusion.
• Apply a tourniquet above the insertion site to impede venous return and prevent further migration of the catheter.
• Arrange for an X-ray, to locate the catheter.

ALLERGIC REACTION

Possible causes
• Hypersensitivity to I.V. solution or additive
Signs and symptoms
• Generalized rash, itching
• Shortness of breath, tachycardia (uncommon)
Intervention
• Notify the doctor.

Continued

I.V. THERAPY

Managing I.V. Therapy Complications
Continued

INFECTION AT INSERTION
SITE

Possible causes
● Poor technique during insertion, cleansing of site, or tubing changes
Signs and symptoms
● Swelling and tenderness at site
Intervention
● Discontinue the infusion.
● Culture the needle or catheter.
● Clean site and apply antimicrobial ointment.
● Cover the site with sterile dressing.

SEPSIS
(usually develops immediately or shortly after the infusion begins)

Possible causes
● Pathogens entering the bloodstream through the I.V. line
Signs and symptoms
● Abrupt rise in temperature, chills
● Nausea and vomiting
● Backache
● Generalized malaise
Intervention
● Discontinue the infusion.
● Culture cannula and samples of solution.
● Record lot number of solution and additives.
● Save remaining solution for lab analysis.
● Notify the doctor immediately.

I.V. THERAPY

Troubleshooting I.V. Flow Rate Deviations

PROBLEM/CAUSE	SOLUTION
Flow rate too fast	
• Patient manipulates the clamp	• Instruct the patient not to touch the clamp, and place tape over it. Restrain the patient or administer the I.V. with an infusion pump or a controller, if necessary.
• Tubing disconnected from the catheter	• Wipe the distal end of the tubing with alcohol, reinsert firmly into catheter hub, and tape at connection site.
• Change in patient position or blood pressure	• Administer the I.V. with an infusion pump or a controller to ensure correct flow rate.
• Positional cannulation	• Manipulate cannula, and place a $2'' \times 2''$ gauze pad under or over the catheter hub to change the angle. Reset the flow clamp at the desired rate. If necessary, remove the cannula and reinsert.
• Flow clamp drifting as a result of patient movement	• Place tape below the clamp.
Flow rate too slow	
• Venous spasm after insertion	• Apply warm soaks over site.
• Venous obstruction from bending arm	• Secure with armboard, if necessary.
• Head pressure change (decreasing fluid in bottle causes solution to run slower due to decreasing pressure)	• Readjust the flow rate.

I.V. THERAPY

Continued

Troubleshooting I.V. Flow Rate Deviations
Continued

PROBLEM/CAUSE	SOLUTION

Flow rate too slow
Continued

• Elevated blood pressure	• Readjust the flow rate. Use an infusion pump or a controller to ensure correct flow rate.
• Change in solution viscosity from medication added	• Readjust the flow rate.
• I.V. container too low or patient's arm or leg too high	• Hang the container higher or remind the patient to keep the arm below heart level.
• Bevel against vein wall (positional cannulation)	• Withdraw the needle slightly or place a folded $2'' \times 2''$ gauze pad over or under the catheter hub to change the angle.
• Excess tubing dangling below insertion site	• Replace the tubing with a shorter piece or tape the excess tubing to the I.V. pole, below the flow clamp (make sure tubing is not kinked).
• Tubing memory (tubing compressed at area clamped)	• Massage or milk the tubing by pinching and wrapping it around a pencil four or five times. Quickly pull the pencil out of the coiled tubing.

I.V. THERAPY

I.V. Fluid Types

The choice of a particular I.V. fluid depends on the patient's normal maintenance requirements, his volume status, and the type of abnormality he has in concentration, composition, or both.

Consider these key points about I.V. fluids:

• *Hypertonic solutions*—those of greater than blood tonicity—are used to replace electrolytes. They're also used to shift extracellular fluid (ECF) from interstices to plasma. When a hypertonic solution is rapidly infused into the body, water will rush out of the cells to the area of greater concentration and the cells will shrivel. Dehydration can also make extracellular fluid hypertonic. Hypertonic solutions should be given slowly to prevent circulatory overload. Commonly used hypertonic solutions include 5% dextrose in 0.9% saline, 5% dextrose in lactated Ringer's, 10% dextrose in water ($D_{10}W$), 20% dextrose in water ($D_{20}W$).

• *Hypotonic solutions* are used to shift plasma into interstitial fluid. When a hypotonic solution surrounds a cell, water will diffuse into the intracellular fluid, causing the cell to swell. Inappropriate use of intravenous fluids or severe electrolyte loss will make body fluids hypotonic. Hypotonic solutions include half-normal saline (0.45% NaCl). For hypernatremia, a hypotonic dextrose infusion may be given.

• *Isotonic solutions* are used to expand ECF volume. When isotonic solutions enter the circulation, they cause no net movement of water across the semipermeable cell membrane. And because the osmotic pressure is the same inside and outside the cells, they do not swell or shrink. Examples of isotonic solutions include normal saline (0.9% NaCl), 5% dextrose in water (D_5W), and lactated Ringer's.

Commonly Infused I.V. Fluids

FLUID TYPE	CALORIES/ LITER	TONICITY
Dextrose in water solutions		
5% dextrose in water	170	Isotonic (252 mOsm/L)
10% dextrose in water	340	Hypertonic (505 mOsm/L)
20% dextrose in water	680	Hypertonic (1,010 mOsm/L)
50% dextrose in water	1,700	Hypertonic (2,525 mOsm/L)
Dextrose in saline solutions		
5% dextrose and 0.2% NaCl	170	Isotonic (320 mOsm/L)
5% dextrose and 0.45% NaCl	170	Hypertonic (406 mOsm/L)
5% dextrose and 0.9% NaCl	170	Hypertonic (559 mOsm/L)
10% dextrose and 0.9% NaCl	340	Hypertonic (812 mOsm/L)
Saline solutions		
0.45% NaCl	0	Hypotonic (154 mOsm/L)
0.9% NaCl	0	Isotonic (308 mOsm/L)
3% NaCl	0	Hypertonic (1,026 mOsm/L)
Multiple electrolyte solutions		
Ringer's solution	0	Isotonic (309 mOsm/L)
Lactated Ringer's solution	9	Isotonic (273 mOsm/L)
5% dextrose in lactated Ringer's	179	Hypertonic (524 mOsm/L)
10% dextrose in lactated Ringer's	349	Hypertonic (776 mOsm/L)

I.V. THERAPY

Administering I.V. Hyperalimentation

The administration of nutrients by the I.V. route can be classified according to the concentration and the extent of nutrients delivered.

I.V. hyperalimentation (IVH) supplies the patient's total energy and nutrient requirements—all necessary proteins, carbohydrates, water, electrolytes, vitamins, trace elements, and fats—exclusively by vein. The hypertonicity of amino acid–glucose solutions necessitates infusion through a central vein; fat emulsion, however, may be infused centrally or peripherally. IVH is indicated when use of the GI tract for nutritional replenishment is inadequate, ill advised, or impossible.

Peripheral parenteral nutrition, a more limited form of nutritional therapy, provides fewer nonprotein calories but greater volume than IVH.

Because IVH fluid has approximately six times the solute concentration of blood, peripheral administration results in sclerosis and thrombosis. To ensure optimal dilution, the superior vena cava—a wide-bore, high-flow vein—must be catheterized.

IVH catheters come in several types. In adults and in children who weigh more than 4.5 kg (10 lb), subclavian venipuncture has been the most commonly used technique for superior vena cava catheterization. Subclavian catheters typically remain in place 30 days or longer.

When cannulation is necessary for longer than 2 months, the doctor will probably implant a silicone rubber, Dacron-cuffed catheter into the jugular, subclavian, cephalic, thyroid, or facial vein, and tunnel it so the catheter exit site is lateral to the xiphoid process. Firm tissue ingrowth into the Dacron cuff, with secondary catheter fixation, occurs in 2 to 3 weeks; the cuff then serves as a mechanical barrier against bacterial and fungal invasion.

Occasionally, the catheter's inserted into the brachial vein in the antecubital fossa or into one of the internal or external jugular veins. However,

Continued

I.V. THERAPY

Administering I.V. Hyperalimentation
Continued

the catheter tip's always positioned in the superior vena cava.

A volumetric infusion pump ensures an accurate, constant flow of IVH fluid. A controller device is not device is not recommended, because the nutrient fluid's viscosity makes consistent flow a problem.

Solution components

IVH solutions, markedly hypertonic (with an osmolarity of 1,800 to 2,400 mOsm/liter), are admixed in the pharmacy under laminar-flow, filtered-air hoods. Usually, 500 ml of dextrose 50% are mixed with 500 ml of 8.5% crystalline amino acid solution, or 350 ml of dextrose 50% are mixed with 750 ml of 5% to 10% protein hydrolysate solution. Electrolytes, vitamins, trace elements, and insulin may be added to the base solution.

Fat emulsions—two or three 500-ml infusions of a 10% or 20% fat emulsion may be given twice weekly to prevent essential fatty acid deficiency in adults.

The isotonicity of fat emulsions permits peripheral administration. However, a 0.22-micron cellulose membrane can't be used for fat emulsion infusion because the fat particles are larger than the filter pores.

When administering fat emulsions, make sure the emulsion's stable and sterile before and during infusion. Never shake the lipid container excessively or use the emulsion if there's any inconsistency in texture or color. During the initial fat infusion, monitor the patient's vital signs as baseline indices. The flow rate should not exceed 1 ml/minute for the first 30 minutes. To minimize the possibility of fat overload or fat embolism, don't administer more than 3 g/kg/day to an adult.

Parenteral Nutrition: Comparing Types

I.V. HYPERALIMENTATION

Solution components/liter
- Dextrose 20% to 25%
- Crystalline amino acids 2.5% to 5%
- Electrolytes, vitamins, trace elements, insulin, and heparin
- Fat emulsion 10% to 20% (usually infused separately)

Uses
- 3 weeks or more (long term)
- For patients with large caloric and nutrient needs
- Provides needed calories; restores nitrogen balance; replaces essential vitamins, electrolytes, minerals, and trace elements
- Promotes tissue synthesis, wound healing, normal metabolic function
- Allows bowel rest and healing; reduces activity in the gallbladder, pancreas, and small intestine

Special considerations
Basic solution
- Nutritionally complete
- Requires minor surgical procedure for central line insertion
- Delivers hypertonic solutions
- May cause metabolic complications

I.V. fat emulsion
- May not be utilized effectively in severely stressed patients
- May interfere with immune mechanisms

PERIPHERAL PARENTERAL NUTRITION

Solution components/liter
- Dextrose 5% to 10%
- Crystalline amino acids 2.75% to 4.25%
- Electrolytes, trace elements, and vitamins
- Fat emulsion 10% or 20% (1 liter dextrose 10% and amino acids 3.5% infused at same time with liter fat emulsion = 1,440 nonprotein calories: 340 from dextrose and 1,100 from fat emulsion)
- Heparin or hydrocortisone as ordered

Uses
- 3 weeks or less
- Maintains nutritional state in patients who can tolerate relatively high fluid volume; those who usually resume bowel function and oral feedings in a few days; and those who are susceptible to catheter-related infections of central venous IVH

Special considerations
Basic solution
- Nutritionally complete for a short term
- Can't be used in nutritionally depleted patients
- Can't be used in volume-restricted patients since higher volumes of solution needed than with central venous IVH

Continued

I.V. THERAPY

Parenteral Nutrition: Comparing Types
Continued

PERIPHERAL PARENTERAL
NUTRITION
Continued

• Doesn't cause patient to gain
weight
• Avoids insertion and maintenance
of central catheter, but patient must
have good veins; I.V. site should be
changed every 48 hours
• Doesn't require surgery for peripheral line insertion
• Delivers less hypertonic solutions than central venous IVH
• May cause phlebitis
• Less chance of metabolic complications than central venous IVH
I.V. fat emulsion
• As effective as dextrose for caloric source
• Diminishes phlebitis if infused at
same time as basic nutrient solution
• Irritates vein in long-term use

PROTEIN-SPARING THERAPY

Solution components/liter
• Crystalline amino acids in same
amounts as IVH
• Electrolytes, vitamins, and min-
erals as ordered
Uses
• 2 weeks or less
• May preserve body protein in a
stable patient
• Augments oral or tube feedings

Special considerations
• Nutritionally incomplete
• Requires little mixing
• May be initiated or stopped at
any point in a patient's hospital
stay
• Other I.V. fluids, medications,
and blood by-products may be
given through same I.V. line
• Not as likely to cause phlebitis
as peripheral parenteral nutrition
• Adds a major expense, with limited benefits

STANDARD I.V. THERAPY

Solution components/liter
• Dextrose, water, and electrolytes in varying amounts
*Examples of frequently used par-
enteral fluids:*
D_5W = 170 calories/liter
$D_{10}W$ = 340 calories/liter
0.9% NaCl (normal saline solution) = 0 calories
• Vitamins as ordered
Uses
• Less than 1 week as nutrition
source
• Maintains hydration (main function)
• Facilitates and maintains normal
metabolic function
Special considerations
• Nutritionally incomplete; does
not administer sufficient calories
to maintain adequate nutritional
status

Troubleshooting Home I.V. Hyperalimentation

Complications, although rare, may develop while the patient undergoes home IVH. Here are signs and symptoms to tell your patient to watch for, and what to do about them:

INFILTRATION

What to watch for
Swelling of tissues around catheter insertion site (shoulder, neck, or arm), discomfort, pain in shoulder or arm on catheter side; swollen tissues cooler than rest of body tissues

What to do
• Call the doctor immediately if you think the catheter has come out of the vein or has ruptured.
• Slow the flow rate if you can't reach the doctor immediately.

CLOUDY SOLUTION OR SEDIMENT IN SOLUTION

What to watch for
Solution cloudy or showing undissolved particles

What to do
• Don't use. Solution may be contaminated. Return solution container to pharmacy at once for exchange.
• If you're mixing your own solution, take extra care with preparation, and don't prepare more than 24 hours' worth of solution at a time.

TOO-RAPID INFUSION

What to watch for
Nausea, headache, lassitude
What to do
• Check to be sure solution is flowing at the rate ordered by your doctor. If you're using an infusion pump, check for mechanical problems.
• If the flow rate is correct and symptoms persist, contact your doctor.

CATHETER DISLODGEMENT

What to watch for
Catheter pulled out of vein
What to do
• Place a sterile gauze pad on insertion site, and apply pressure.
• Notify your doctor.

CRACK OR BREAK IN CATHETER TUBING

What to watch for
Fluid leaking out through crack or break in tubing
What to do
• Apply padded hemostat above break, to prevent entry of air.
• Call your doctor at once.

Continued

I.V. THERAPY

Troubleshooting Home I.V. Hyperalimentation
Continued

CLOTTED CATHETER

What to watch for
Solution flow stops and doesn't
enter the vein
What to do
• Notify doctor. He may instill
streptokinase or heparin into the
catheter to try to dissolve clot.

HYPERGLYCEMIA (high blood sugar)

What to watch for
Fatigue, restlessness, confusion,
anxiety, weakness, urine tests positive for sugar; in severe cases, possibly delirium and/or coma
What to do
• Notify doctor at once.

PHLEBITIS

What to watch for
Pain, tenderness, skin redness,
and warmth
What to do
• Rest, and apply gentle heat to
the site. Elevate your arm if the
catheter is inserted in your arm.
• Relief should occur within 24 to
72 hours, and condition should
subside within 3 to 5 days.

• Notify your doctor immediately.
He may want to examine you or
give you additional care instructions.

INFECTION

What to watch for
Fever (body temperature above
37.8° C. [100° F.]), redness and/or
pus at insertion site
What to do
• Notify your doctor so he can determine the fever's source.
• If infection is present, the doctor
will remove the catheter to have
the tip cultured.

AIR EMBOLISM

What to watch for
Apprehension, chest pain, rapid
heartbeat, low blood pressure resulting in dizziness and fainting,
bluish appearance; problem
caused by air entering catheter,
usually during bottle changes
What to do
• Call your doctor immediately. If
symptoms are severe, go to hospital
emergency department at once.
• Lie on your left side, with your
head slightly lower than the rest
of your body.

I.V. THERAPY

Guide to Major Blood Components

WHOLE BLOOD

Description
Blood complete with all plasma and cell constituents
Indications
• To restore adequate blood volume in hemorrhaging, trauma, or burn patients
Contraindications
• When the patient doesn't need volume increase and a specific component is available
Cross matching
Necessary
Shelf life
• 21 days at 5° C. (41° F.)
Administration techniques
• Straight line set, Y-set, or microaggregate recipient set
Special considerations
• Although whole blood is seldom transfused, necessary components are extracted from it.
• Plasma protein fraction or normal serum albumin given as volume expander until patient's component needs are known.

RED BLOOD CELLS
(packed, frozen)

Description
Whole blood with 80% of the supernatant plasma removed
Indications
• To correct red blood cell deficiency and improve oxygen-carry-

ing capacity of blood
• To transfuse organ transplant patients or to treat repeated febrile transfusion reactions (frozen-thawed RBCs)
Contraindications
• When the patient's anemic from a deficiency of the hematopoietic nutrients; for example, iron, vitamin B_{12}, or folic acid
• When the patient's asymptomatic, but his hematocrit level must be raised
Cross matching
Necessary
Shelf life
• For stored fresh packed cells, 21 days; or 24 hours after opening
• For stored frozen cells, 3 years; or 24 hours after thawing
Administration techniques
• Straight line set, Y-set, or microaggregate recipient set
Special considerations
• RBCs have the same oxygen-carrying capacity as whole blood without overload hazards. Their use avoids buildup of potassium and ammonia that can occur in stored blood plasma. Frozen-thawed RBCs are expensive.

WHITE BLOOD CELLS
(leukocyte concentrate)

Description
Whole blood with RBCs and 80% of supernatant plasma removed
Continued

I.V. THERAPY

Guide to Major Blood Components
Continued

WHITE BLOOD CELLS
Continued

Indications
● To treat life-threatening granulo-cytopenia from intensive chemo-therapy
Contraindications
● When the patient's health de-pends on the recovery of bone marrow functions
Cross matching
Must be ABO compatible
Shelf life
● 24 hours after collection at 5° C. (41° F.)
Administration techniques
● Straight line set with standard in-line filter. Dosage: 1 unit daily until infection clears
Special considerations
● *Important:* Infusion induces fe-ver and can cause mild hyperten-sion, severe chills, disorientation, and hallucinations.

PLASMA
(fresh, fresh-frozen)

Description
Uncoagulated plasma separated from whole blood
Indications
● To treat a clotting factor defi-ciency, hypovolemia, or severe hepatic disease
● To prevent dilutional hypocoa-gulability

Contraindications
● When blood coagulation can be corrected with available specific therapy
Cross matching
Unnecessary
Shelf life
● For fresh plasma, within 6 hours after collection
● For fresh-frozen plasma, 12 months at − 18° C. (− 0.2° F.); or 2 hours after thawing
Administration techniques
● Any straight line set; administer as rapidly as possible.
Special considerations
● Normal saline solution not needed for Y-set because the component contains no RBCs.

PLATELETS

Description
Platelet sediment from platelet-rich plasma, resuspended in 30 to 50 ml of plasma
Indications
● To treat thrombocytopenia when bleeding is caused by decreased platelet production, increased platelet destruction, functionally abnormal platelets, or massive transfusions of stored blood
Contraindications
● When bleeding's unrelated to decreased number of platelets or abnormal function of platelets
Continued

Guide to Major Blood Components
Continued

PLATELETS
Continued

Cross matching
Unnecessary (donor plasma and recipient's RBCs should be ABO compatible)
Shelf life
• Up to 72 hours after whole blood collection
Administration techniques
• Syringe or component drip set only; give as rapidly as possible
• Must use a nonwettable filter
• Dosage: 2 units/kg of body weight raise platelet count at least 50,000/mm³
Special considerations
• Usually given when platelet count is below 10,000/mm³

PLASMA PROTEIN FRACTION

Description
5% selected proteins solution pooled plasma in buffered, stabilized saline diluent
Indications
• To treat hypovolemic shock or hypoproteinema
Contraindications
• When the patient has severe anemia or heart failure
Cross matching
Unnecessary
Shelf life
• 5 years if refrigerated; 3 years at room temperature

Administration techniques
• Any straight line set; rate and volume depend on the patient's condition and response.
Special considerations
• Don't mix in same line with protein hydrolysates and alcohol solutions.

NORMAL SERUM ALBUMIN 5% OR 25%

Description
Heat-treated, aqueous, chemically processed fraction of pooled plasma
Indications
• To treat shock
• To prevent marked hemoconcentration
• To maintain electrolyte balance
• To treat hypoproteinemia
Contraindications
• When the patient has severe anemia or heart failure
Cross matching
Unnecessary
Shelf life
• 5 years at 2° C. (35.6° F.); 3 years at room temperature
Administration techniques
• Give undiluted, or diluted with saline solution or D_5W.
• In hypoproteinemia: administer slowly (1 to 3 ml/min) to prevent rapid volume expansion.
Special considerations
• Can't transmit hepatitis

I.V. THERAPY

Administering Blood: Some Important Guidelines

When you administer blood, always follow hospital policy and procedure. But keep these important guidelines in mind as well:

• Carefully compare patient and donor unit identification. If your patient's hemorrhaging, you may not want to spend time checking identification numbers. However, skipping this step could result in a serious transfusion reaction. Most hemolytic transfusion reactions associated with ABO mismatching stem from identification errors.

• Always administer blood through a filter that removes cellular debris (preferably a microaggregate filter). Cellular debris in donor blood includes leukoagglutinins, which react with the recipient's leukocytes to form a white cell aggregate that becomes trapped in pulmonary microcirculation. This promotes pulmonary congestion with resistance to forward blood flow into the left atrium. The resulting sluggish blood flow may lead to pulmonary edema and poor alveolar gas exchange. Expect such signs and symptoms as respiratory distress, cyanosis, fever, chills, and, eventually, hypotension.

• Always use normal saline solution to prime the tubing. Never mix a drug or another solution with blood. Once you begin the transfusion, monitor the patient for signs and symptoms of immediate transfusion reaction: fever, chills, hypotension, chest and lumbar pain, nausea, vomiting, wheal formation, eyelid edema, bronchospasm, hives, and itching.

• Check the patient's temperature and vital signs before you start the transfusion. Notify the doctor of any temperature elevation and note any increase from baseline during transfusion. Such an increase may indicate transfusion reaction. Document baseline hemodynamic parameters, breath sounds, and urine output and quality.

Continued

I.V. THERAPY

Administering Blood: Some Important Guidelines
Continued

• Warm banked blood to body temperature (98.6° F. [37° C.]) before administration. Consider this step essential for massive transfusions (replacement of 50% or more of the patient's blood volume at one time or replacement of the patient's total blood volume within 24 hours). Exchange transfusions and potent cold agglutinins also require warming. Banked blood—stored at 33° to 43° F. (1° to 6° C.)—may cause hypothermia if administered without warming. Hypothermia increases the ventricular fibrillation risk, impairs the patient's ability to withstand further blood loss, and promotes metabolic acidosis. Warm banked blood with an electric blood warmer, if available—this automatically heats blood to body temperature. *Never* warm blood above body temperature or above 107° F. (42° C.) because excessive warming causes hemolysis. (If possible, avoid using a blood-warming coil that you must immerse in warm water. This system takes too long in an emergency and may lead to hemolysis.)

• Provide psychological support. The patient and his family may react to the prospect of a blood transfusion with both relief (because it's a life-saving measure) and fear (because they perceive it as a last-ditch effort). They may also worry about the possibility of disease transmission (especially acquired immunodeficiency syndrome or hepatitis) from donor blood. Some patients may refuse transfusions on religious or cultural grounds. Explain all procedures, and reassure the patient and his family.

I.V. THERAPY

Recognizing Transfusion Reactions

During a blood transfusion, your patient's at risk for developing any of five types of reactions. To learn to recognize them and to intervene appropriately, study this chart.

If your patient develops any sign or symptom of a reaction, immediately follow this procedure:
- Stop the transfusion.
- Change the I.V. tubing to prevent infusing any more blood. Save the tubing and blood bag for analysis.
- Administer saline solution I.V. to keep the vein open.
- Take the patient's vital signs.
- Notify the doctor.
- Obtain urine and blood samples from the patient and send them to the laboratory.
- Prepare for further treatment.

HEMOLYTIC

Signs and symptoms
Include chills, fever, low back pain, headache, chest pain, tachycardia, dyspnea, hypotension, nausea and vomiting, restlessness, anxiety, shock

Special considerations
- Expect to place the patient in a supine position, with his legs elevated 20° to 30°, and to administer oxygen, fluids, and epinephrine to correct shock.

- Expect to administer mannitol to maintain the patient's renal circulation.
- Expect to insert an indwelling (Foley) catheter to monitor the patient's urinary output (should be about 100 ml/hr).
- Expect to administer antipyretics to lower the patient's fever. If his fever persists, expect to apply a hypothermia blanket or to give tepid sponge or alcohol baths.

Continued

Recognizing Transfusion Reactions
Continued

PLASMA PROTEIN INCOMPATIBILITY

Signs and symptoms
Include chills, fever, flushing, abdominal pain, diarrhea, dyspnea, hypotension

Special considerations
• Expect to place the patient in a supine position, with his legs elevated 20° to 30°, and to administer oxygen, fluids, and epinephrine to correct shock.
• Expect to administer corticosteroids.

BLOOD CONTAMINATION

Signs and symptoms
Include chills, fever, abdominal pain, nausea and vomiting, bloody diarrhea, hypotension

Special considerations
• Expect to administer fluids, antibiotics, corticosteroids, vasopressors, and a fresh transfusion.

FEBRILE

Signs and symptoms
Range from mild chills, flushing, and fever to extreme signs and symptoms resembling a hemolytic reaction

Special considerations
• Expect to administer an antipyretic and an antihistamine for a *mild* reaction.
• Expect to treat a *severe* reaction the same as a hemolytic reaction.

ALLERGIC

Signs and symptoms
Range from pruritus, urticaria, hives, facial swelling, chills, fever, nausea and vomiting, headache, and wheezing to laryngeal edema, respiratory distress, and shock

Special considerations
• Expect to administer parenteral antihistamines or, for a severe reaction, epinephrine or corticosteroids.
• If the patient's only sign of reaction is hives, expect to restart the infusion, as ordered, at a slower rate.

I.V. THERAPY

Administering Plasma and Plasma Fractions

PLATELETS

Administration method
Component drip set or component syringe set with a nonwettable filter
Usual administration rate
Rapidly, 1 unit/10 min
Complications
Hepatitis, allergic reaction, febrile reaction, circulatory overload

PLASMA, FRESH FROZEN PLASMA

Administration method
Plasma administration set, standard blood administration set with a standard blood filter (microaggregate recipient set unnecessary)
Usual administration rate
1 unit in less than 1 hour for hypovolemia
Complications
Hepatitis, allergic reaction, febrile reaction, circulatory overload

PLASMA PROTEIN FRACTION

Administration method
Standard blood administration set with a standard blood filter (microaggregate recipient set unnecessary)
Usual administration rate
Usually 5 to 10 ml/min, depending on patient's condition and response
Complications
Circulatory overload, hypotension

ALBUMIN

Administration method
Albumin administration set (supplied by manufacturer)
Usual administration rate
Rapidly for shock; 5 to 10 ml/min for hypoproteinemia
Complications
Circulatory overload, pyrogenic reaction, microbial contamination, hepatitis (uncommon)

Continued

Administering Plasma and Plasma Fractions
Continued

CRYOPRECIPITATE

Administration method
Component drip set or component syringe set
Usual administration rate
Rapidly, 10 ml/min
Complications
Hepatitis

FACTOR VIII CONCENTRATE

Administration method
Plastic syringe for I.V. injection; plastic syringe and infusion set (provided by manufacturer) for I.V. infusion
Usual administration rate
10 to 20 ml/3 min
Complications
Hepatitis

PROTHROMBIN COMPLEX

Administration method
Standard blood administration set with filter
Usual administration rate
Varies greatly but usually 1 vial/5 min
Complications
Hepatitis (very high risk)

GAMMA GLOBULIN

Administration method
I.M. injection
Usual administration rate
Not applicable
Complications
Allergic reaction, especially in the patient with anti-IgA antibody

I.V. THERAPY

Pediatric Calculations

Before giving any drug, you're responsible for determining whether or not the dose and dosage are safe for your patient. If you're unsure, follow these guidelines.

To check the prescribed *dose* (the amount of drug given at one time), use one of the formulas below. If the result of your calculation differs significantly from the prescribed dose, withhold the drug and check with the doctor or pharmacist.

Young's rule:

$$\frac{\text{adult dose} \times \text{child's age (in years)}}{\text{child's age} + 12} = \text{dose}$$

Clark's rule:

$$\frac{\text{adult dose} \times \text{child's weight (in pounds)}}{150} = \text{dose}$$

Fried's rule
(for a child less than age 1):

$$\frac{\text{adult dose} \times \text{child's age (in months)}}{150} = \text{dose}$$

Surface area rule:

$$\frac{\text{adult dose} \times \text{surface area of child (in square meters)}}{1.7} = \text{dose}$$

Note: Use a body surface area nomogram to determine surface area.

Now, suppose you question the prescribed *dosage.* As you know, dosage includes the prescribed dose, the frequency of administration, and the number of doses to be given. To check dosage, you must consult a drug reference book or the pharmacist. Always double-check the dose and dosage for a potent drug with another nurse.

Administering Oral Medications: Important Guidelines

Because of their different physical and mental make-ups, children require special care. So, when giving them medication, keep these guidelines in mind:
• DO get acquainted with your patient before approaching him with the medication. Use a matter-of-fact but friendly manner to put him at ease. Act as though you expect his cooperation.
• DO check the patient's identification band, and observe the Five Rights of medication administration.
• DO find out if he has a nickname and use it, if it makes him feel more comfortable.
• DO check any medication that's unfamiliar to you, and any dose or dosage that seems inappropriate for your patient. Have a second nurse check dose and dosage for potent medications, such as insulin, anticoagulants, and digitalis preparations. Call the pharmacist if you have any questions.
• DON'T try to trick a child

into taking his medication. Doing so may make him less cooperative the next time he has to take it, and will make him distrust nurses.
• DO encourage your patient's cooperation by acting as if you expect it. Praise him for cooperating, if he does.
• DO give an older child choices, if possible, to give him some feeling of control over his care. For example, offer him a choice of beverage to take with (or after) his medication.
• DON'T threaten, insult, or embarrass your patient.
• DON'T tell the child the medication's candy, because he may try to take more than the prescribed dosage. Or, he may not trust you.
• DON'T leave any unattended medications at your patient's bedside.
• DON'T let the medication cart or tray out of your sight while administering medications. Your patient may try to take something from it while you're not looking.

Continued

Administering Oral Medications: Important Guidelines
Continued

• DO allow the child to become familiar with the oral administration device. For example, if you administer the medication in a soufflé cup, give him a chance to play with one.

• DON'T give the child a chewable tablet if he has loose teeth.

• DO explain the relationship between illness and treatment to an older child. He may be more cooperative if he realizes the medication will help him.

• DON'T insist that your patient swallow his medication or attempt to hold his nose or mouth shut to force him to swallow it. Doing so may cause him to choke.

• DO administer medications to an infant in a manner similar to the feeding activity. By giving medications through a nipple, for example, you take advantage of the infant's natural sucking reflex.

• DO try to comfort an infant while administering the medication, to calm him.

• DO place a tablet or capsule near the back of your patient's tongue, and give him plenty of water or flavored drink to help him swallow it.

• DO encourage the child to tip his head slightly forward, not back, when swallowing a tablet or capsule. Throwing his head back increases the risk of aspiration. Make sure he swallows the medication.

• DO try allowing parents to administer the oral medication to a difficult patient. But check your hospital's policy first.

• DO observe the child closely to see if the medication has the intended effect or any adverse effects on him.

• DO note any special considerations on your patient's Kardex; for example, "Jason will take his tablet only if it's crushed and mixed with a flavoring syrup."

• DO document carefully on the medication record all medications that you administer.

SPECIAL CONSIDERATIONS

Administering Medications to Elderly Patients

If you're providing drug therapy for elderly patients, you'll want to understand patterns of drug use in the elderly, age-related pharmacokinetic and physiologic changes that may alter drug dosage, how to improve compliance in the elderly, and common adverse reactions.

Medication consumption patterns

The elderly consume more prescription and nonprescription drugs than the young because they have a greater variety of diseases requiring one or more medications. Besides major diseases, elderly persons may take medication for aches and pains, constipation and other GI complaints, insomnia, and various skin disorders.

An older person's socioeconomic status, personal health, and health care environment (extended-care facility or community living, for example) may affect his drug use. And his doctors and nurses have an influence as well, particularly in regard to p.r.n. medications.

In addition, institutionalized elderly patients take more medications than outpatients.

Physiologic changes affecting drug action

As a person ages, gradual changes occur in his anatomy and physiology. Some of these

changes may alter the therapeutic and toxic effects of medications.
Body composition
Proportions of body fat, lean tissue, and water change with age. Total body mass and lean body mass tend to decrease; the proportion of body fat tends to increase. Although varying from person to person, these changes affect the relationship between a drug's concentration and solubility in the body.

For example, a *water-soluble* drug is distributed mostly to the aqueous body parts and to lean tissue. Since the elderly person has less lean tissue for the drug to be distributed to, more of the drug remains in the bloodstream. This may result in increased blood concentration unless the drug dosage is reduced.

The distribution of *fat-soluble* drugs may also be affected by age-related changes in body composition. As the proportion of body fat increases, fat-soluble drugs must be distributed to a greater tissue volume. Accordingly, this increased volume may initially lower blood drug concentrations; however, after the body fat is saturated with drug, it may store the drug and slowly release it back into the general circulation, thus increasing the drug's duration of action.

Continued

Administering Medications to Elderly Patients
Continued

GI function
In the elderly, decreases in gastric acid secretion and GI motility slow emptying of stomach contents and movement of intestinal contents through the entire tract. Furthermore, although inconclusive, research shows the elderly may have more difficulty absorbing medications.

Hepatic function
Although significantly reduced hepatic function normally isn't associated with the aging process, the liver's ability to metabolize certain drugs does decrease with age. Decreased hepatic function may cause:
• more intense drug effects, from higher blood levels
• longer-lasting drug effects, from prolonged blood concentrations
• greater incidence of drug toxicity.

Patient noncompliance
Noncompliance with prescribed drug therapy is a major problem in the elderly. It includes:
• failure to take prescribed doses
• consumption of inappropriate doses
• failure to follow the correct schedule
• premature discontinuance of medications

• consumption of medications prescribed for previous disorders
• indiscriminate use of medications ordered p.r.n.

The following factors may contribute to noncompliance:
• *Hearing loss.* This can prevent the elderly patient from hearing instructions completely and correctly. As a result, he may take a drug dose at the wrong time or in the wrong way.
• *Loss of visual acuity* and the ability to discriminate colors, as well as glare from eyeglasses. This can interfere with the patient's ability to comply. Vision problems limit his ability to read instructions, differentiate among pills and capsules, or spot drug deterioration.

Note: Patients see reds and yellows best, blues and greens the worst.
• *Decreased muscle strength and coordination,* as well as arthritic joints. This can make removing bottle caps difficult or impossible.
• *Financial limitations.* If your elderly patient is on a fixed income, he may try to make his medications last longer by skipping doses or prolonging dosage intervals. And he may fail to refill prescriptions.

Common Adverse Reactions

The elderly reportedly have twice as many adverse drug reactions as younger people. This increased incidence stems from greater drug consumption, poor compliance, and physiologic changes.

Signs and symptoms of adverse drug reactions—confusion, weakness, and lethargy—may be mistakenly attributed to senility or disease. If the adverse reaction isn't identified, the patient may continue to receive the drug. Furthermore, he may receive unnecessary additional medication to treat complications caused by the original medication.

When caring for elderly patients, stay particularly alert for toxicities resulting from diuretics, digoxin, corticosteroids, sleep medications, and nonprescription drugs.

• *Diuretic toxicity*
The use of potassium-wasting diuretics, such as hydrochlorothiazide and furosemide, may result in fluid and electrolyte imbalance in the elderly patient. Because average total body water decreases with age, normal doses of these drugs may result in fluid loss and even dehydration in an elderly patient. These diuretics may deplete serum potassium, causing weakness; and they may raise blood uric acid and glucose levels, complicating preexisting gout and diabetes mellitus.

• *Digoxin toxicity*
As the body's renal function and excretion rate decline, serum digoxin concentrations may build to toxic levels, causing nausea, vomiting, diarrhea, and, most serious, cardiac dysrhythmias. If your patient can't speak or has lost his hearing or sight, he may not be able to convey his symptoms to you. Therefore, observe him for changes in appetite, orientation, and mood.

• *Corticosteroid toxicity*
Corticosteroids, such as prednisone, may also cause
Continued

SPECIAL CONSIDERATIONS

Common Adverse Reactions
Continued

adverse reactions in the elderly. Short-term effects include fluid retention and psychological manifestations ranging from mild euphoria to acute psychotic reactions. Long-term toxic effects, such as osteoporosis, can be especially severe in elderly patients who have been taking prednisone or related steroidal compounds for months or even years. Observe your patient for subtle changes in appearance, mood, and mobility, as well as for signs of impaired healing and fluid and electrolyte disturbances.

• *Sleep medication toxicity*
In some cases, sedatives or sleeping aids cause excessive sedation or residual drowsiness. Consequently, elderly patients may fall or injure themselves. To help prevent serious injury to elderly patients taking sedatives or sleeping aids, institute precautionary measures, such as raising bed side rails whenever necessary.

• *Nonprescription drug toxicity*
Although prescription drugs are more commonly recognized as the cause of adverse drug reactions, nonprescription drugs also can cause significant problems for the elderly.

• *Aspirin and aspirin-containing analgesics,* among the nonprescription drugs most commonly purchased by the elderly, have minimal toxicity when used in moderation. But prolonged ingestion may cause GI irritation and gradual blood loss resulting in severe anemia.

• *Laxatives and cathartics* may cause the following problems:
—diarrhea, if an elderly patient's extremely sensitive to a laxative such as bisacodyl
—lipid pneumonia from chronic oral use of mineral oil as a lubricating laxative, if the patient aspirates small residual oil droplets in his mouth.

When Your Patient's a Stroke Victim

If your patient's ability to swallow is seriously impaired, giving oral medication isn't safe. But what if he's a stroke patient and only one side of his head and body is affected? If he's alert and cooperative, with your help he may be able to swallow oral medication.

Before you begin, remember that your patient's stroke has probably affected him in many ways. Keep this in mind when you give him his medication. For example, if the vision on his impaired side is affected, approach and treat him from his unimpaired side, so he can see what you're doing. If he suffers from some form of aphasia, speak to him slowly, explaining the procedure to him in words he can understand.

Try to give him the medication in solid form, because a textured substance is easier for him to control than a liquid. Crush uncoated tablets or open soft capsules, and mix them with a soft food, like applesauce or mashed potatoes. However, never mix the medication with a milk product. Milk products will stimulate salivation, which will increase the risk of aspiration.

Tip: If your patient's afraid of choking on his medication, place the fingers of his unimpaired

hand on his neck. When he feels his neck muscles working as he swallows, his confidence may be restored. To be perfectly safe, however, have suctioning equipment handy.

Minimize the risk of aspiration in any stroke patient by following this procedure:

● When you're giving him medication or food, put it on the back of his tongue, on the *unimpaired* side of his mouth. Then, gently turn his head toward the unimpaired side. *Important:* Never tilt his head backward. This position makes aspiration more likely.

● Give him a sip of water and ask him to swallow. At the same time, press lightly on the *impaired* side of his neck, to stimulate the swallowing reflex. Continue to give him small sips of water until he's swallowed the food or medication. Then, check his mouth. Remove any food or medication trapped on his impaired side.

● Finally, document the entire procedure. Record foods that seem to give your patient particular trouble.

As always, use your own judgment. If you think giving oral medication's too risky for your patient, tell the doctor. He may choose another route.

Drugs and the Pregnant Patient

To safely and beneficially administer drugs to a pregnant patient, you must first understand the special nature of the maternal/fetal twosome. Several major physiologic changes occur in a pregnant woman that can interfere with drug action. A woman's blood and plasma volume increase, resulting in a reduced serum albumin level. Less albumin available to bind drugs that enter the maternal system means more unbound, or free, drug available to cross the placenta to the fetus.

In addition, the pregnant woman's hepatic blood flow decreases, so her liver metabolizes drugs more slowly than usual. Consequently, the transfer of unmetabolized drugs from mother to fetus occurs over a longer period, thus prolonging the drug's effect on the fetus.

Renal blood flow and glomerular filtration *increase* during pregnancy, causing the mother's kidneys to excrete drugs more rapidly. As a result, you must carefully monitor drug dosage.

The placenta's role. Before a drug can reach the fetus, it must first cross the placental membrane. This usually occurs by simple drug diffusion.

Once a drug crosses the placenta and enters fetal circulation, it does one of two things, depending on its composition. Most drugs travel through the umbilical and portal veins to the fetal liver, where they're converted and detoxified. Other drugs pass through the liver to the ductus venosus and inferior vena cava to the heart, which distributes the drugs to the brain and coronary arteries. Then, more than half the blood and drug combination travels back through the umbilical arteries, crosses the placenta, and reenters maternal circulation. The remaining drug-laden blood continues to circulate in the fetus.

The fetus excretes the drug mainly through its kidneys. However, because excretion's slow, drugs may accumulate in the fetus.

The fetus also excretes a small drug amount through its lungs, sweat glands, and bile into the amniotic fluid. Because the fetus swallows the amniotic fluid, the excreted drugs are reabsorbed into the fetal circulation. Drug therapy in a pregnant patient must be closely correlated with fetal gestational age. Whether a particular drug adversely affects the fetus depends on the stage of fetal growth and development at the time of drug exposure. The first and third trimesters warrant the most serious consideration, since the fetus is most vulnerable to drug effects at these times.

Continued

Drugs and the Pregnant Patient
Continued

During these times, give *all* drugs with extreme caution. The most sensitive period is the first trimester, when fetal organs are differentiating. During this time, withhold *all* drugs unless doing so would jeopardize the mother's health.

At birth, the newborn must rely on his own metabolism to excrete any drug remaining in his body. Since his detoxifying systems are not fully developed, any residual drug may take a long time to be metabolized—and thus may induce prolonged toxic reactions. Consequently, drugs should be used with caution during the last 3 months of pregnancy and only when absolutely necessary at term.

Nevertheless, in many circumstances, pregnant women must continue to take certain drugs. In such cases, the potential risk to the fetus is outweighed by the mother's need for the drug.

To avoid adverse drug effects in your pregnant patient, follow these guidelines:
• Before administering any drug to a woman of childbearing age, ask the date of her last menstrual period and whether she could possibly be pregnant.
• Avoid administering all drugs except those essential to maintain the pregnancy or the mother's health. Be particularly cautious during the first and third trimesters when the fetus is most vulnerable.
• Apply topical drugs cautiously. Many topically applied drugs can be absorbed in amounts large enough to harm the fetus.

As a precaution, remind your pregnant patient to check with her doctor before taking any drug. *Remember:* Alcohol and caffeine are drugs, too. Caution your pregnant patient to use them judiciously.

If your patient plans to breast-feed, advise her that most drugs a nursing mother takes appear in breast milk. Drug levels in breast milk tend to be high when blood levels are high—generally, shortly after taking each dose. Therefore, advise the mother to breast-feed *before* taking medication, not *after*.

Breast-feeding should be temporarily interrupted and replaced with bottle-feeding when the mother must take:
• tetracyclines
• chloramphenicol
• sulfonamides (during first 2 weeks postpartum)
• oral anticoagulants
• iodine-containing drugs
• antineoplastics
• propylthiouracil.

Handling Antineoplastic Drugs Safely

Most antineoplastic drugs are highly toxic compounds that cause mutagenic, carcinogenic, or teratogenic effects. Some antineoplastic drugs are hazardous on direct contact, causing skin, eye, and mucous membrane irritation, or even tissue ulceration and necrosis. This toxicity causes potential hazards for doctors, pharmacists, and nurses during preparation and administration of parenteral antineoplastic drugs.

The following guidelines are adapted from recommendations developed by the National Institutes of Health. Review them in light of your own institution's protocol.

To prepare parenteral antineoplastic drugs:

• Perform all procedures in a Class II vertical laminar flow biological safety cabinet, if available. If you must use a horizontal flow cabinet, turn off the fan before starting drug preparation. If your facility doesn't have a biological safety cabinet, prepare these drugs on a clean table or countertop in a quiet area with no air turbulence.

• Cover the work surface with plastic-backed absorbent paper. Change the paper and wipe the work area thoroughly with 70% alcohol, using a disposable towel, after any spills and after each work shift.

• Before beginning drug preparation procedures, put on surgical gloves and a surgical gown with knit cuffs. After preparing the drugs, remove and replace overtly contaminated gloves or gowns.

• Vent vials containing reconstituted drugs to reduce internal pressure.

• Wrap a sterile, alcohol-dampened cotton swab around the needle and vial top as you withdraw the needle from the vial septum. Similarly, place an alcohol-dampened swab at the needle tip when ejecting air bubbles from a filled syringe.

• Wipe the external surfaces of syringes and I.V. bottles clean of any drug contamination.

• When breaking the top off a glass ampul, wrap the ampul neck at the anticipated break point with a sterile, alcohol-dampened cotton swab to contain the aerosol produced.

Continued

Handling Antineoplastic Drugs Safely
Continued

• Make sure you properly identify and date all syringes and I.V. bottles containing antineoplastic drugs.
• When disposing of contaminated needles and syringes, keep them intact to prevent aerosol generation created by clipping needles. Place them in a leakproof and puncture-resistant container. Then place this container, as well as any contaminated items, in an appropriately labeled, plastic bag–lined box for incineration. Washable gowns may be laundered normally.
• Dispose of waste antineoplastic drugs in accordance with federal and state requirements applicable to toxic chemical waste; check your institution's protocol for specific procedures.
To administer parenteral antineoplastic drugs:
• Put on a protective outer garment. Wear disposable surgical gloves during any procedures that may entail drug leakage.
• When removing bubbles from syringes or I.V. tubing, carefully place a sterile, alcohol-dampened cotton swab over the tips of needles, syringes, or I.V. tubing to collect any drug discharge.
• Dispose of contaminated needles and syringes intact. Place them in a leakproof and puncture-resistant container, and follow the steps outlined above for disposing of contaminated equipment and waste antineoplastic drugs after preparation.
• Avoid skin contact and minimize aerosol generation when handling the excreta of patients who've received antineoplastic drugs; wear disposable surgical gloves and follow standard and approved disposal procedures.

General precautions
• In case of skin contact with an antineoplastic drug, thoroughly wash the affected area with soap and water. Flush affected eyes with copious amounts of clean water for at least 15 minutes; then seek medical attention.
• Wash your hands thoroughly after preparing or administering any antineoplastic drug.

Using I.V. Controllers and Pumps

Controllers and pumps electronically regulate the flow of I.V. solution or drugs when extreme accuracy of administration is required. Controllers regulate gravity flow by counting drops and achieve the desired infusion rate by compressing the I.V. tubing. However, because controllers simply count drops, which aren't always of equal size, these devices don't achieve the accuracy of volumetric pumps, which measure flow rate in milliliters per hour.

Volumetric pumps, used for high-pressure drug infusion or for accurate delivery of fluids or drugs, have mechanisms to propel the solution at the desired rate under pressure. The peristaltic pump applies pressure to the I.V. tubing to force the solution through it. (Not every peristaltic pump is volumetric; some count drops.) The piston-cylinder pump, called a volumetric pump, pushes the solution through special disposable cassettes. The portable syringe pump, another volumetric pump type, delivers small fluid amounts over a long duration.

Both controllers and pumps have various detectors and alarms that automatically signal or respond to an infusion's completion, air in line, low battery power, and occlusion or inability to deliver at the set rate. Depending on the problem, these devices may sound or flash an alarm, shut off, or switch to a keep-vein-open rate.

Follow these guidelines when using I.V. controllers and pumps:

To set up a controller, attach the controller to the I.V. pole. Then, insert the administration set spike into the I.V. container and fill the drip chamber no more than halfway to avoid miscount of the drops. Rotate the chamber so the fluid touches all sides to remove any vapor that could interfere with correct counting. Now, prime the tubing and clamp it closed. Position the drop sensor above the fluid level in the drip chamber and below the drop port to ensure correct drop counting. Insert the tubing into the controller, close the door, and completely open the flow clamp.

Continued

Using I.V. Controllers and Pumps
Continued

To set up a volumetric pump, attach the pump to the I.V. pole. Then, insert the administration set into the I.V. container spike, and completely fill the drip chamber to prevent air bubbles from entering the tubing. Next, prime the tubing and clamp it closed. Now, follow the manufacturer's instructions for tubing placement.

To set up a nonvolumetric peristaltic pump, follow the steps for setting up a controller.

● Position the controller or pump on the same side of the bed as the I.V. or anticipated venipuncture site to avoid crisscrossing I.V. lines over the patient.

● Plug in the machine and attach its tubing to the needle or catheter hub. If you're using a controller, position the drip chamber 30″ (76 cm) above the infusion site to ensure accurate gravity flow.

● Depending on the machine, set the appropriate dials on the front panel to the desired infusion rate and volume. Always set the volume dial 50 ml less than the prescribed volume or 50 ml less than the volume in the container, so you can hang a new container before the old one empties completely. Then, turn on the machine and press the start button.

● Check I.V. line patency and watch for infiltration. If you're using a controller, monitor infusion rate accuracy.

● Turn on the alarm switches. Then, explain the alarm system to the patient to prevent apprehension when a change in the infusion activates the alarm.

Special considerations
● Frequently monitor the pump or controller and the patient to ensure the device's correct operation and maintenance of the prescribed flow rate and to detect infiltration and such complications as infection and air embolism.

Using a Volume-Control I.V. Set

A volume-control set—an I.V. line with a chamber—delivers precise fluid amounts and, when the fluid's exhausted, prevents air from entering the I.V. line. This device is especially useful for continuous infusion of fluids or medication in children or for intermittent infusion of medication to adults already receiving I.V. therapy.

All models of volume-control sets consist of a graduated chamber (120 to 250 ml), with a spike and filtered air line on its top and administration tubing underneath.

Follow these guidelines when using a volume-control I.V. set:
• Remove the volume-control set from its box, and close all the clamps.
• Remove the guard from the volume-control set spike, insert the spike into the I.V. solution container, and hang the container on the I.V. pole.
• Open the air vent clamp. Then, open the lower clamp on the I.V. tubing and slide it

upward until it's positioned slightly below the drip chamber. Next, close the clamp.
• If you're using a volume-control set with a hinged latex valve or floating latex diaphragm, open the upper clamp until the fluid chamber fills with about 30 ml of solution. Then, close the clamp and carefully squeeze the drip chamber until it's half full.

If you're using a volume-control set with a membrane filter, open the upper clamp until the fluid chamber fills with about 30 ml of solution, and then close the clamp. Open the lower clamp, and squeeze the drip chamber flat with two fingers of your opposite hand. If you squeeze the drip chamber with the lower clamp closed, you'll damage the membrane filter. Keeping the drip chamber flat, close the lower clamp. Now, release and reshape the drip chamber, so it fills halfway.
• Open the lower clamp, prime the tubing, and close

Continued

Using a Volume-Control I.V. Set
Continued

the clamp. To use as a primary line, insert adapter into the catheter of needle hub. To use as a secondary line, attach a needle to the adapter on the volume-control set. Wipe the Y-injection port of the primary tubing with an alcohol sponge, and insert the needle. Then, tape the connection.

• To add medication, wipe the injection port on the volume-control set with an alcohol sponge, and inject the medication. Place a label on the chamber, indicating the drug, dosage, and date.

• Open the upper clamp, fill the fluid chamber with the prescribed amount of solution, and close the clamp. Gently rotate the chamber to mix the medication.

• Open the lower clamp on the volume-control set, and adjust the drip rate as ordered. After the infusion's completed, open the upper clamp and let 10 ml of I.V. solution flow into the chamber and through the tubing to flush them.

• If you're using the volume-control set as a secondary I.V. line, close the lower clamp and reset the flow rate on the primary line. If you're using the set as a primary I.V. line, close the lower clamp, refill the chamber to the prescribed amount, and begin the infusion again.

Special considerations

• If you're using a membrane filter set, avoid administering suspensions, emulsions, blood, or blood components through it.

• If you're using a latex diaphragm set, the diaphragm may stick after repeated use. If it does, close the air vent and upper clamp, invert the drip chamber, and squeeze it. If the diaphragm opens, re-open the clamp and continue to use the set.

• If the drip chamber of a hinged latex valve or floating latex diaphragm set overfills, immediately close the upper clamp and air vent, invert the chamber, and squeeze excess fluid from the drip chamber back into the graduated chamber.

Some Common Drugs of Abuse: Effects

As you can see in the chart, these drugs may cause physical or psychological dependence, or both. *Physical dependence* (or addiction) occurs when a person's body gets so accustomed to the drug that he cannot function normally without it. When the drug is withheld, physical and psychic withdrawal symptoms develop. A person may inadvertently become physically addicted, for example, when he takes certain drugs for a long-term illness.

Psychological dependence (or habituation) produces a desire to take drugs to feel good. The user has no physical compulsion to continue taking the drug. He may merely want to escape problems or situations he can't cope with, or he may seek pleasure and want to stimulate his senses.

Drug tolerance occurs when the user needs to take larger and larger doses to achieve the same effects. Accurate determination of tolerance levels is important in treatment programs.

CATEGORY/DRUG	POSSIBLE EFFECTS
Narcotics codeine heroin hydromorphone meperidine methadone morphine	Euphoria; respiratory depression; constricted pupils; nausea, risk of infection and hepatitis from I.V. (mainlined) drugs; wan, undernourished appearance; drowsiness and lethargy—user is on the "nod" (alternately dozing and waking) **Overdose:** Slow, shallow breathing; clammy skin; convulsions; coma; possibly death **Withdrawal:** Watery eyes, runny nose, yawning, anorexia, irritability, tremors, panic, chills and sweating, dilated pupils, piloerection (gooseflesh), cramps, nausea

Continued

SPECIAL CONSIDERATIONS

Some Common Drugs of Abuse: Effects
Continued

CATEGORY/ DRUG	POSSIBLE EFFECTS

Stimulants
amphetamine
cocaine
methylphenidate
phenmetrazine

Increased wakefulness, excitation, euphoria, talkativeness, irritability, dilated pupils, nervousness, increased pulse rate, elevated blood pressure
Overdose: Agitation, fever, hallucinations, convulsions, possibly death
Withdrawal: Apathy, long periods of sleep, irritability, depression, disorientation

---

Depressants
barbiturates
chloral hydrate
glutethimide
methaqualone
other depressants

Extreme drowsiness; slurred speech; disorientation; drunken behavior without alcohol use; slow, rapid, or shallow breathing; constricted pupils
Overdose: Shallow breathing; cold, clammy skin; dilated pupils; weak, rapid pulse; coma; possibly death
Withdrawal: Anxiety, insomnia, tremors, delirium, convulsions, possibly death

---

benzodiazepines   No significant effects

Guide to Selected Drug Toxicities

Drug toxicity follows overdose or ingestion of a drug meant for external use. Cumulative toxicity may result from long-term use of a slowly-excreted drug. The information that follows tells you how to identify, treat, and reverse toxic reactions with specific antidotes and how to relieve their symptoms with other drugs or with supportive measures. Generally, the doses cited are recommended for adults. With some exceptions, children's doses should be calculated individually.

ACETAMINOPHEN

Signs and symptoms to watch for:
• In the first 3 to 4 hours after ingestion: nausea, vomiting, anorexia, and sweating (some patients have no symptoms)
• 24 to 36 hours after ingestion: patient may still be asymptomatic; liver enzyme levels may begin to rise.
• Hepatic toxicity may develop 2 to 5 days after ingestion. Watch for vomiting, right upper quadrant tenderness, elevated SGOT, SGPT, and serum bilirubin levels, increased prothrombin time (PT) and possible hypoglycemia.

How to confirm toxicity:
• Monitor SGOT, SGPT, and serum bilirubin levels, and PT.
• Monitor serum acetaminophen levels. Levels over 300 mcg/ml 4 hours after ingestion suggest severe hepatic damage; levels under 120 mcg/ml 4 hours after ingestion rarely indicate hepatic damage.

What to do:
• Stop drug.

• Induce emesis with ipecac syrup or do gastric lavage.
Important: Don't give ipecac syrup if the patient's unconscious.
• Supportive measures include parenteral fluids, fresh frozen plasma, or clotting factors.
• Immediately begin therapy with acetylcysteine (Mucomyst), the direct antidote to acetaminophen overdose. Acetylcysteine solution may be diluted to a 5% concentration with a soft drink to make it more palatable.

BARBITURATES

Signs and symptoms to watch for:
(All indicate acute toxicity)
CNS: headache, confusion, ataxia, CNS depression ranging from sleepiness to coma (may be preceded by excitement and hallucinations)
CV: hypotension
EENT: ptosis, miosis, mydriasis in severe poisoning
Skin: cyanosis, especially in ear lobes, nose, or fingers; occasional blisters or bullous lesions

Continued

Guide to Selected Drug Toxicities
Continued

BARBITURATES
Continued

Other: slow, shallow breathing; flaccid muscles; hypothermia, hyperthermia; shock.

How to confirm toxicity:
• Positively identify ingested drug.
• Measure and identify barbiturates in blood, urine, or gastric contents.
• Monitor for potentially lethal blood levels:
—phenobarbital, 80 mcg/ml or higher
—amobarbital and butabarbital, 50 mcg/ml or higher
—secobarbital and pentobarbital, 30 mcg/ml or higher.

What to do:
• Stop drug.
• Maintain adequate airway.
• Maintain adequate oxygen intake and carbon dioxide removal.
• Begin gastric lavage (most effective when started within 2 hours of ingestion).
• Delay absorption with activated charcoal.
• Barbiturate toxicity has no specific antidote. Don't give analeptic drugs such as caffeine.
• Maintain blood pressure by infusing 5% plasma or low–molecular weight dextran I.V. Monitor central venous pressure. If fluid infusion doesn't maintain blood pressure, give metaraminol or norepinephrine.
• Elevate patient's head 15 degrees to help prevent cerebral edema.
• Give up to 40 ml/kg fluids daily if renal function is adequate. Maintain daily urine output at 15 to 30 ml/kg.
• Monitor sodium, potassium, and chloride levels daily.
• In phenobarbital toxicity, forced alkaline diuresis with sodium bicarbonate and osmotic diuretic may be useful.
• Treat hypothermia by applying blankets. Avoid too-rapid warming.
• Dialysis is indicated in severe barbiturate poisoning or inadequate renal function.
• Frequently monitor patient's pulse rate, temperature, skin color, reflexes, and response to painful stimuli.

CARDIOTONIC GLYCOSIDES
(for example, digitalis leaf, digitoxin, digoxin)

Signs and symptoms to watch for:
CNS: headache, weakness, fatigue, somnolence, dizziness, ataxia, confusion, aphasia, paresthesias, seizures, coma, apathy, depression, restlessness, insomnia, giddiness, excitement, agitation, delusions, hallucinations, psychosis

Continued

SPECIAL CONSIDERATIONS

Guide to Selected Drug Toxicities
Continued

CARDIOTONIC GLYCOSIDES
Continued

CV: premature ventricular beats (most common in adults), paroxysmal and nonparoxysmal junctional rhythms, atrioventricular dissociation; paroxysmal atrial tachycardia with AV block (most common in children)
Other: anorexia, nausea, vomiting, blurred vision, yellow cast to vision or halos around lights, diarrhea
How to confirm toxicity:
● Monitor EKG.
● Monitor blood levels: 2.5 ng/ml of digoxin and 35 ng/ml of digitoxin may indicate toxicity.
What to do:
● Stop drug.
● Treat dysrhythmias. If patient has marked hypokalemia and atrial, junctional, or ventricular tachycardia, give potassium chloride.

   If patient isn't hypokalemic, use phenytoin. If phenytoin's contraindicated, infuse lidocaine as an I.V. bolus, followed by constant infusion.

   In patients with atrial tachycardia with AV block and premature ventricular contractions, give propranolol by slow I.V. infusion. The patient with second- or third-degree AV block, SA block, and marked sinus bradycardia may

need an artificial pacemaker.
● Monitor EKG.

NARCOTICS
(for example, codiene, hydromorphone, morphine, opium alkaloids, and meperidine)

Signs and symptoms to watch for:
CNS: respiratory depression; apnea; CNS depression, ranging from stupor to profound coma; muscle tremors and twitches; delirium; disorientation; hallucinations; and (with meperidine derivatives) seizures
CV: bradycardia, hypotension, cyanosis, and (with meperidine derivatives) possible tachycardia
EENT: miosis (with morphine derivatives and methadone), mydriasis (with meperidine derivatives)
GI: dry mouth (with meperidine derivatives)
Other: cold, clammy skin; hypothermia; and flaccid skeletal muscles.
Confirming diagnostic measures:
● Make a positive identification of ingested drug, if possible.
● Note symptoms:
—coma, pinpoint pupils, and depressed respirations indicating

Continued

Guide to Selected Drug Toxicities
Continued

NARCOTICS
Continued

morphine derivative and methadone toxicity. Keep in mind that in
terminal narcosis or severe hypoxia, morphine and methadone
toxicity may cause mydriasis.
—coma, dilated pupils, depressed
respirations indicating meperidine
derivative toxicity.
• Analyze urine, blood, gastric
contents, or all three fluids for
narcotics.
What to do:
• Stop drug.
• Establish airway; ventilate as
needed.
• Induce emesis with ipecac
syrup or do gastric lavage, especially within first 2 hours of ingestion.
Important: Do not give ipecac
syrup if patient's unconscious or
shows signs of CNS depression.
• Give naloxone (Narcan).
• Keep in mind that a narcotic an-
tagonist may precipitate acute
withdrawal syndrome in patients
physically addicted to narcotics.
• Maintain body warmth.
• Maintain adequate fluid intake.
• Treat shock with oxygen, I.V.
fluids, and vasopressors as
needed.
• Monitor vital signs and level of
consciousness frequently.

SALICYLATES

*Signs and symptoms to watch
for:*
• Mild toxicity—burning pain in
mouth, throat, or abdomen; slight
to moderate hyperpnea; lethargy;
vomiting; tinnitus; hearing loss;
and dizziness
• Moderate toxicity—ecchy-
moses, restlessness, incoordina-
tion, dehydration, fever, sweating,
delirium, excitability, marked lethargy, and severe hyperpnea
• Severe toxicity—sodium, potassium, and bicarbonate loss and
metabolic acidosis in young children; coma; convulsion; cyanosis;
oliguria; uremia; pulmonary
edema; respiratory failure; and
severe hyperpnea
*Confirming diagnostic mea-
sures:*
• Monitor blood salicylate levels
for 6 hours after ingestion. (*Note:*
Salicylamide isn't determined by
serum salicylate analysis.) Look
for the following salicylate levels
in adults:
—mild intoxication: 45 to 65 mg/dl
—moderate intoxication: 65 to 90
mg/dl
—severe intoxication: 90 to 120
mg/dl
Blood levels of 120 mg/dl or more
are usually fatal.

Continued

Guide to Selected Drug Toxicities
Continued

SALICYLATES
Continued

• Blood levels may continue to rise for 6 to 10 hours after overdose.
What to do:
• Stop drug.
• Induce emesis with ipecac syrup.
Important: Don't give ipecac syrup if patient's unconscious.
• If patient shows CNS depression, do gastric lavage and protect airway.
• Delay absorption with activated charcoal.
• Give a saline cathartic.
• For hypotension, give I.V. fluids according to patient's acid/base and electrolyte status.
• For respiratory depression, give artificial respiration with oxygen.
• For hypoglycemia, give dextrose I.V.
• Maintain fluid balance with dextrose 5% in water with sodium chloride.
• For acidosis, give sodium bicarbonate by slow I.V. infusion over 24 to 48 hours.
• For bleeding from hypoprothrombinemia, give phytonadione (vitamin K_1), I.M. or I.V.
• For impaired renal function, use dialysis to remove salicylates.
• For hyperpyrexia, sponge patient with tepid water. Don't use alcohol.
• Continue monitoring serum sodium, potassium, glucose, blood gases, and salicylate levels.

SPASMOLYTICS
(for example, aminophylline, papaverine, and theophylline)

Signs and symptoms to watch for:
CNS: headache, insomnia, irritability, restlessness, convulsions, hyperreflexia, coma
CV: tachycardia, marked hypotension
EENT: tinnitus and flashing lights
GI: nausea, vomiting, epigastric pain, hematemesis, and diarrhea
Skin: cyanosis
Other: dehydration, extreme thirst, tachypnea, respiratory arrest, and fever
What to do:
• Stop drug.
• Induce emesis with ipecac syrup or do gastric lavage.
Important: Do not give ipecac syrup if the patient's unconscious.
• Delay absorption with activated charcoal.
• Give I.V. fluids and oxygen and use additional supportive measures to prevent hypotension and maintain fluid and electrolyte balance.
• Monitor serum levels until drug concentration is below 20 mcg/ml.

Detecting Drug Interactions

On the following pages, you'll find drugs causing significant interactions. They're grouped by major drug category; for example, *Anti-infectives*.

By using these charts, you can determine if the drugs your patient is taking have the potential to interact—and how to intervene if they do.

If a drug you're checking isn't listed, the reason may be that no well-substantiated and clinically significant drug interactions occur. But double-check by also looking up the drug's major category. In drug classes containing many individual drugs, we've specifically named only those that are most frequently ordered. Interactions, however, commonly involve all members of the drug class.

Analgesics: Interactions affecting therapy

Salicylates interact adversely with many drugs, including warfarin. Because salicylates are highly protein-bound, they can displace warfarin from its protein-binding sites. The result: more warfarin in the bloodstream and an intensified anticoagulant effect. Similarly, if a patient takes aspirin while also taking probenecid for gout, he may get little gout relief. In continuous, low doses, aspirin has an antagonistic effect on the uric acid excretion that probenecid normally stimulates.

SALICYLATES

All salicylates: aspirin, choline magnesium, trisalicylate, choline salicylate, magnesium salicylate, salsalate, sodium salicylate, sodium thiosalicylate

Interacting drug
• Antacids (in large doses)
• Corticosteroids
Possible effect
Decreased salicylate effectiveness from hastened salicylate excretion
Special considerations
• Warn the patient against taking large doses of antacids.

Interacting drug
• Probenecid
• Sulfinpyrazone
Possible effect
Gout from increased serum uric acid levels; interaction blocks uric acid excretion

Continued

Detecting Drug Interactions
Continued

SALICYLATES
Continued

Interacting drug
● Probenecid
● Sulfinpyrazone
Possible effect
Gout from increased serum uric acid levels; interaction blocks uric acid excretion
Special considerations
● Monitor serum uric acid levels and assess the patient for signs and symptoms of gout.
● Instruct the patient to avoid over-the-counter products containing aspirin. Also advise him to avoid alcohol and foods high in purine, such as coffee.

NARCOTICS, OPIOID ANALGESICS, AND PROPOXYPHENE
All narcotics and opioid analgesics: alphaprodine, butorphanol, codeine, fentanyl, hydrocodone, hydromorphone, levorphanol, meperidine, methadone, morphine, nalbuphine, opium, oxycodone, oxymorphone, pentazocine

Possible effect
Additive respiratory depression
Special considerations
● As ordered, give a lower dose of the narcotic analgesic (when administered with or a few hours before the barbiturate anesthetic).
● Monitor the patient's respiratory rate.

MEPERIDINE

Interacting drug
● Phenytoin
Possible effect
Meperidine toxicity from increased meperidine metabolism resulting in formation of normeperidine, a potentially toxic metabolite
Special considerations
● Monitor the patient for signs of normeperidine toxicity, such as CNS excitation (tremors or twitches).
● Decrease the meperidine dosage, as ordered.

Anti-Infectives: Interactions Affecting Therapy

Drug interactions involving aminoglycosides can be among the most serious. These drugs can impair kidney function and hearing, even when used alone. If you must administer an aminoglycoside with another drug that's nephrotoxic or ototoxic, such as cephalothin or a loop diuretic, make sure you monitor the patient frequently for signs and symptoms of renal failure or hearing loss.

If your patient is just beginning anti-infective therapy while still receiving another drug, observe him closely for an acute initial reaction. For example, if you give erythromycin to a patient who's already receiving theophylline, watch for theophylline toxicity.

AMINOGLYCOSIDES
All aminoglycosides: amikacin, gentamicin, kanamycin, neomycin, netilmicin, streptomycin, tobramycin

Interacting drug
• Loop diuretics (ethacrynic acid, furosemide, and bumetanide)

Possible effect
Ototoxicity from increased antibiotic concentration in ear fluid (a synergistic effect); interaction also has the additive effect of increasing the ototoxicity of both drugs

Special considerations
• Monitor the patient for hearing loss. If possible, make sure that baseline audiometric testing is done and that testing is repeated once or twice weekly during therapy.
• Regularly check the patient's hearing with a tuning fork, if available.
• Teach the patient to recognize and report signs and symptoms of ototoxicity.
• Regularly document hearing assessments.

Interacting drug
• Neuromuscular blocking agents (nondepolarizing muscle relaxants, such as tubocurarine, atracurium, and pancuronium)

Possible effect
Neuromuscular blockade and respiratory arrest from additive or synergistic neuromuscular blocking activity

Continued

Anti-Infectives: Interactions Affecting Therapy
Continued

AMINOGLYCOSIDES
Continued

Special considerations
• Use these drugs together cautiously if the patient's renal or hepatic function is impaired.
• Reduce the dosage frequency of the neuromuscular blocking agent, as ordered, according to the patient's response.
• Monitor the patient for apnea.
• Perform a baseline lung assessment by checking lung sounds and the rate, rhythm, and depth of respirations.
Interacting drug
• Penicillins, especially carbenicillin (mixed in the same I.V. solution)
Possible effect
Failure to eliminate infection. When an aminoglycoside is mixed with high concentrations of a penicillin (especially carbenicillin) in an I.V. solution, the aminoglycoside becomes inactive.
Special considerations
• Don't mix aminoglycosides and penicillins together in the same I.V. container. Instead, give the drugs 1 hour apart. *Note:* In patients with impaired renal function, these drugs may interact despite this precaution. Monitor for decreased therapeutic effect.

CEPHALOSPORINS
All cephalosporins: for example, cefoperazone, cefamandole, moxalactam

Interacting drug
• Alcohol
Possible effect
Antabuse-like reaction from inhibition of an enzyme called aldehyde dehydrogenase, causing acetaldehyde accumulation. *Note:* Other cephalosporins don't cause this interaction.
Special considerations
• Teach the patient to recognize signs and symptoms of Antabuse-like reaction: sweating, diarrhea, nausea and vomiting, and headache.
• Instruct him to avoid alcohol, including over-the-counter drugs containing alcohol (for example, liquid cough and cold preparations).

Continued

Anti-Infectives: Interactions Affecting Therapy
Continued

PENICILLINS
All penicillins: for example, ampicillin, cloxacillin, penicillin G

Interacting drug
- Probenecid

Possible effect
High plasma penicillin levels from decreased renal excretion of the anti-infective

Special considerations
- A penicillin may be given with probenecid to achieve higher plasma penicillin levels.
- Carefully document the patient's fluid intake and output.
- Use cautiously if the patient has impaired renal function.

Ampicillin

Interacting drug
- Allopurinol

Possible effect
Rash or other hypersensitivity reaction; mechanism unknown. *Note:* Other penicillins don't cause this interaction.

Special considerations
- Monitor the patient for rash or other hypersensitivity reaction.

TETRACYCLINES
All tetracyclines: for example, doxycycline, oxytetracycline, tetracycline

Interacting drug
- Antacids containing aluminum, calcium, or magnesium
- Iron salts

Possible effect
Decreased absorption of tetracycline from chelation (combination of tetracycline and metal)

Special considerations
- Don't give tetracycline and an antacid simultaneously. Instead, give tetracycline 1 hour before the antacid or 2 hours after the antacid.
- Instruct the patient not to take tetracycline with milk or milk-containing products and to avoid iron supplements.

OTHER ANTI-INFECTIVES

Amphotericin B
Interacting drug
- Corticosteroids
- Diuretics

Possible effect
Hypokalemia from additive effects

Continued

Anti-Infectives: Interactions Affecting Therapy
Continued

OTHER ANTI-INFECTIVES
Continued

Special considerations
• Obtain baseline serum potassium levels before therapy begins. Then, monitor serum levels at least twice weekly, especially if the patient's receiving a digitalis glycoside.
• Check serum potassium levels before giving diuretic doses.
• Assess the patient for signs and symptoms of hypokalemia.
• Encourage him to consume foods and beverages high in potassium, such as bananas and fruit juices.

Erythromycin
Interacting drug
• Theophylline
Possible effect
Theophylline toxicity from decreased theophylline metabolism
Special considerations
• Regularly monitor plasma theophylline measurements and report rising levels. Therapeutic levels range from 10 to 20 mcg/ml; higher levels may be toxic.

• Assess the patient for signs and symptoms of theophylline toxicity.
• Warn the patient not to take any other drugs, including over-the-counter drugs, without the doctor's approval.

Isoniazid
Interacting drug
• Carbamazepine
Possible effect
Increased toxicity of both drugs from a mutual synergism that produces a double-drug interaction
Special considerations
• Monitor the patient for increased liver enzymes, a sign of isoniazid toxicity.
• Monitor for carbamazepine toxicity and increased plasma carbamazepine levels. Toxic levels are greater than 10 mcg/ml (or as specified in your hospital's laboratory manual). Signs and symptoms of toxicity include dizziness, ataxia, stupor, and nausea and vomiting.

Note: Carbamazepine toxicity may cause bone marrow depression.

Anticonvulsants: Interactions Affecting Therapy

The most important point to remember when administering anticonvulsants is that these drugs have a very narrow therapeutic index. A small dosage increase can cause drug toxicity, while a small decrease can render the drug ineffective. And when you consider that many other drugs can interfere with the metabolism of an anticonvulsant, you can see why you'll need to monitor your patient very closely if he's receiving an anticonvulsant with another drug.

ALL ANTICONVULSANTS

Interacting drug
• Phenothiazines
• Tricyclic antidepressants
Possible effect
Increased risk of seizures from lowered seizure threshold
Special considerations
• Take seizure precautions.
• Monitor the patient for development of seizures.
• Adjust anticonvulsant dosage, if ordered.

CARBAMAZEPINE

Interacting drug
• Phenobarbital
Possible effect
Increased risk of seizures from increased carbamazepine metabolism

Special considerations
• Monitor plasma carbamazepine levels. Therapeutic levels range from 3 to 9 mcg/ml.
Interacting drug
• Erythromycin
• Propoxyphene
Possible effect
Carbamazepine toxicity from inhibition of carbamazepine metabolism
Special considerations
• Monitor plasma carbamazepine levels.
• Adjust carbamazepine dosage, if ordered.

PHENOBARBITAL

Interacting drug
• Valproic acid

Continued

Anticonvulsants: Interactions Affecting Therapy
Continued

PHENOBARBITAL
Continued

Possible effect
Phenobarbital toxicity; valproic acid inhibits phenobarbital metabolism.

Special considerations
• Observe the patient for signs and symptoms of phenobarbital toxicity, such as sedation and drowsiness.
• Monitor plasma phenobarbital levels. Therapeutic levels range from 15 to 40 mcg/ml.

PHENYTOIN

Interacting drug
• Chloramphenicol, isoniazid, trimethoprim, and sulfonamides
• Cimetidine
• Disulfiram

Possible effect
Phenytoin toxicity from blocked metabolism of phenytoin

Special considerations
• Monitor plasma phenytoin levels. Therapeutic levels range from 10 to 20 mcg/ml.

• Check the patient for signs and symptoms of phenytoin toxicity, such as nystagmus and ataxia.
• Monitor liver function test results for signs of hepatic damage.
• Adjust phenytoin dosage, as ordered.

Interacting drug
• Folic acid

Possible effect
Increased risk of seizures because folic acid increases phenytoin's metabolism and interferes with phenytoin's absorption

Special considerations
• Avoid this combination, if possible. If the drugs must be given together, increase the phenytoin dosage, as ordered.
• Monitor plasma phenytoin levels. Therapeutic levels range from 10 to 20 mcg/ml.
• Take seizure precautions and observe the patient for signs and symptoms of phenytoin toxicity, such as nystagmus and ataxia.

Oral Anticoagulants: Interactions Affecting Therapy

When administering oral anti-coagulants, keep these points in mind:

• If your patient is taking warfarin concurrently with such drugs as phenylbutazone, quinidine, or cimetidine, monitor his prothrombin time as ordered and check for signs and symptoms of bleeding. These drugs tend to enhance warfarin's anticoagulant effect. *Important:* If necessary, remind the doctor to order routine prothrombin values.

• Warn your patient to avoid taking salicylates (and over-the-counter preparations containing them) while on warfarin therapy, unless the doctor specifically approves this combination.

• Monitor the patient's hemoglobin and hematocrit values. A decrease may mean bleeding.

• Watch for signs of occult bleeding: melena, cloudy urine, or coffee-ground vomitus.

WARFARIN AND DICUMAROL

Interacting drug
• Alcohol
Possible effect
Bleeding from additive hypo-prothrombinemic effect or decreased anticoagulant effect from enhanced warfarin metabolism
Special considerations
• Watch for bleeding and signs of occult bleeding.
• Instruct him to avoid alcoholic beverages in excess. Over-the-counter products containing alcohol, such as liquid cough and cold preparations, can be used with caution.

Interacting drug
• Salicylates
Possible effect
Bleeding from displacement of warfarin from protein-binding sites and from additive hypoprothrombinemic effect
Special considerations
• Monitor prothrombin time.
• Monitor the patient's hemoglobin and hematocrit values. A decrease in these values may indicate bleeding.

Continued

SPECIAL CONSIDERATIONS

Oral Anticoagulants: Interactions Affecting Therapy
Continued

WARFARIN AND DICU-
MAROL
Continued

• Watch for bleeding and
signs of occult bleeding.
• Instruct the patient to avoid
aspirin and over-the-counter
products containing aspirin.
• Tell him to report excessive
or unexplained bleeding or
bruising to his doctor.
Interacting drug
• Carbamazepine, barbitu-
rates, or rifampin
Possible effect
Decreased anticoagulant ef-
fect from enhanced warfarin
or dicumarol metabolism
Special considerations
• Monitor prothrombin time.
• Watch for signs of in-
creased clotting effect.
• Adjust anticoagulant dos-
age, as ordered.
Interacting drug
• Phenylbutazone, oxyphen-
butazone, or chloral hydrate
Possible effect
Bleeding from displacement
of warfarin or dicumarol from
protein-binding sites
Special considerations
• Use extreme caution when

giving any of these drugs
with an oral anticoagulant.
• Monitor prothrombin time.
• Watch for bleeding and
signs of occult bleeding.
• Notify the doctor if the patient develops GI distress or
other signs that might indicate bleeding.
Interacting drug
• Acetaminophen
Possible effect
Bleeding if the patient takes
more than 2.8 g of acetaminophen daily for more than 2
consecutive weeks; mecha-
nism unknown
Special considerations
• If the patient is taking acetaminophen continuously at
high doses, monitor his prothrombin time and watch for
bleeding and signs of occult
bleeding.
• Check the combination
drug products your patient's
taking, especially analgesics,
for acetaminophen.
    Note: This interaction isn't
significant if acetaminophen
is taken only in the usual
dosages recommended for
relief of fever or pain.

SPECIAL CONSIDERATIONS

Oral Antidiabetics: Interactions Affecting Therapy

When teaching your patient about oral antidiabetic drugs, stress these points:
• Warn him about the risks of drinking alcohol-containing beverages; he may be setting himself up for an Antabuse-like reaction. Oral antidiabetic drugs alter alcohol metabolism and cause acetaldehyde accumulation.
• Remind him that many over-the-counter cough and cold preparations contain alcohol. Tell him to check product labels and to avoid products containing alcohol.
• Advise him to wear a Medic Alert tag identifying his condition and the medication he takes.

ORAL ANTIDIABETICS
All orally administered antidiabetics: for example, acetohexamide, chlorpropamide, tolazamide, and tolbutamide

Interacting drug
• Alcohol
Possible effect
Antabuse-like reaction from acetaldehyde accumulation;
also, possible hypoglycemia from additive effect
Special considerations
• Instruct the patient to avoid alcohol and over-the-counter products containing alcohol (for example, liquid cough and cold preparations).
• Teach him to recognize the symptoms of an Antabuse-like reaction: sweating, diarrhea, nausea and vomiting, and headache.
Interacting drug
• Beta blockers; for example, propranolol, nadolol, pindolol, and timolol
Possible effect
Hypoglycemia without the usual signs and symptoms. Beta blockers inhibit hypoglycemic signs and symptoms mediated by the adrenergic nervous system and may block rebound glycogenolysis.
Special considerations
• Monitor serum glucose levels regularly.
• Instruct the patient to adhere to his prescribed diet.
• To minimize this interaction, the doctor may order a cardioselective beta blocker,
Continued

Oral Antidiabetics: Interactions Affecting Therapy
Continued

ORAL ANTIDIABETICS
Continued

such as atenolol or metoprolol.
Interacting drug
• Rifampin
Possible effect
Hyperglycemia and poor control of diabetes from increased metabolism of antidiabetic drug
Special considerations
• Monitor serum glucose levels.
• Test urine for glucose and acetone regularly.
• Check the patient for signs and symptoms of hyperglycemia: anorexia, nausea and vomiting, lethargy, thirst, and polyuria.
Interacting drug
• Sulfonamides
Possible effect
Hypoglycemia, mainly from displacement of antidiabetic drug from protein-binding sites
Special considerations
• Monitor serum glucose levels.
• Observe the patient for

signs and symptoms of hypoglycemia: sweating, confusion, pallor, and hunger.
Interacting drug
• MAO inhibitors
• Salicylates (in high doses)
Possible effect
Hypoglycemia; mechanism unknown
Special considerations
• Monitor serum glucose levels.
• Observe the patient for signs and symptoms of hypoglycemia: sweating, confusion, pallor, and hunger.
Interacting drug
• Thiazide diuretics
Possible effect
Thiazide-produced hyperglycemia, which antagonizes antidiabetic action
Special considerations
• Monitor serum glucose levels.
• Test urine for glucose and acetone regularly.
• Observe the patient for signs and symptoms of hyperglycemia: anorexia, nausea and vomiting, lethargy, thirst, and polyuria.

SPECIAL CONSIDERATIONS

Cardiovascular Drugs: Interactions Affecting Therapy

Of all cardiovascular drugs, antihypertensives are probably the most widely used. These drugs are commonly prescribed in combinations of two or more to take advantage of each drug's different mechanism of action. The intended therapeutic result is an increased antihypertensive effect with minimal adverse reactions. Unfortunately, antihypertensives may interact adversely with many other drugs, complicating drug therapy.

If your patient's receiving a beta blocker while taking an antidiabetic medication, monitor his serum glucose levels. Beta blockers can mask the normal signs and symptoms of hypoglycemia.

The calcium channel blockers verapamil, nifedipine, and diltiazem have become increasingly important in the treatment of angina and dysrhythmias. Of the three drugs, verapamil is most likely to cause dangerous interactions. Consult this chart for details on these and other cardiovascular drugs.

ANTIARRHYTHMICS

Lidocaine
Interacting drug
● Disopyramide or phenytoin
Possible effect
Myocardial depression, congestive heart failure, and dysrhythmias from additive effect
Special considerations
● Observe the patient for signs and symptoms of myocardial depression (such as hypotension and bradycardia), congestive heart failure, and dysrhythmias.
● Obtain regular EKG readings, as ordered.

Interacting drug
● Beta adrenergic blockers or cimetidine
Possible effect
Lidocaine toxicity from inhibited lidocaine metabolism
Special considerations
● Observe the patient for signs and symptoms of lidocaine toxicity, such as sedation, confusion, and seizures.
● Also check for signs and symptoms of myocardial depression (such as hypotension and bradycardia), congestive heart failure, and dysrhythmias.
● Monitor plasma lidocaine levels.
Interacting drug
● Cimetidine

Continued

Cardiovascular Drugs: Interactions Affecting Therapy
Continued

ANTIARRHYTHMICS
Continued

Possible effect
Quinidine toxicity from inhibited quinidine metabolism
Special considerations
• Monitor plasma quinidine levels. Therapeutic levels range from 1 to 6 mcg/ml.
• Regularly check the patient's pulse and blood pressure.
• Monitor his EKG readings for widening QRS complex and dysrhythmias.
• Adjust quinidine dosage, if ordered.
Interacting drug
• Barbiturates
• Phenytoin
• Rifampin
Possible effect
Decreased quinidine effect from increased quinidine metabolism
Special considerations
• Monitor plasma quinidine levels. Therapeutic levels range from 1 to 6 mcg/ml.
• Regularly check the patient's pulse and blood pressure.
• Monitor his EKG readings for widening QRS complex and dysrhythmias.
• Assess the effectiveness of quinidine therapy.

ANTIHYPERTENSIVES
All antihypertensives causing orthostatic hypotension: for example, sympatholytic drugs

Interacting drugs
• Phenothiazines; for example, chlorpromazine and prochlorperazine
• Nitrates; for example, nitroglycerin and isosorbide dinitrate
Possible effect
Orthostatic hypotension from additive hypotensive effect
Special considerations
• Monitor the patient for orthostatic changes in blood pressure and pulse while he's lying, sitting, and standing.
• Advise the patient to stand slowly to avoid dizziness.
• Administer nitrates while the patient is lying down to avoid severe headache and symptomatic hypotension.
Captopril
Interacting drug
• Potassium or potassium-sparing diuretics (spironolactone, triamterene, and amiloride)
Possible effect
Hyperkalemia from potassium retention caused by captopril
Special considerations
• Regularly monitor serum potas-
Continued

Cardiovascular Drugs: Interactions Affecting Therapy
Continued

ANTIHYPERTENSIVES
Continued

sium and other electrolyte levels.
• Monitor EKG readings for widening of QRS complexes, tall T waves, and ventricular fibrillation.
• Check for other signs and symptoms of hyperkalemia: irritability, nausea, and diarrhea.
Clonidine
Interacting drug
• Levodopa
Possible effect
Reduced antiparkinsonian effectiveness from negation of levodopa activity
Special considerations
• Check for signs and symptoms of parkinsonism: facial grimacing, jerky arm and leg movements, and bobbing head.
• As ordered, gradually discontinue clonidine over 24 hours and replace with another antihypertensive drug.
Interacting drug
Tricyclic antidepressants
Possible effect
Decreased antihypertensive effectiveness; mechanism unknown
Special considerations
• Monitor the patient's blood pressure carefully.
• Emphasize the importance of having his blood pressure

checked regularly after he leaves the hospital.
• Adjust the clonidine dosage, as ordered.
Prazosin
Interacting drug
• Beta adrenergic blockers
Possible effect
Acute hypotension from synergistic increase in prazosin effects
Special considerations
• Monitor the patient carefully for acute hypotension, especially following the first prazosin dose. First dose should be given at bedtime.
• Emphasize the importance of having his blood pressure checked regularly after he leaves the hospital.

BETA ADRENERGIC BLOCKERS
All beta adrenergic blockers: atenolol, metoprolol, nadolol, pindolol, propranolol, timolol

Interacting drug
• All bronchodilators; for example, albuterol, aminophylline, metaproterenol, terbutaline, and theophylline
Possible effect
Bronchospasm and wheezing from antagonistic action of beta blocker

SPECIAL CONSIDERATIONS

Continued

Cardiovascular Drugs: Interactions Affecting Therapy
Continued

BETA ADRENERGIC BLOCKERS
Continued

Special considerations
• Check the patient's history for asthma.
• Monitor him for signs and symptoms of pulmonary disorders: wheezing, shortness of breath, restlessness, increased pulse rate, thready pulse, and dizziness.
• Instruct the patient to report breathing problems, and warn him not to stop taking the drug without consulting the doctor.
• To minimize this interaction, the doctor may order a cardioselective beta blocker, such as atenolol or metoprolol.

CALCIUM CHANNEL BLOCKERS
All calcium channel blockers: diltiazem, nifedipine, verapamil

Interacting drug
• Beta blockers
Possible effect
Heart block from negative inotropic effect of both agents. *Note:* This interaction is somewhat more significant with verapamil.
Special considerations
• Observe the patient for signs

and symptoms of congestive heart failure, such as shortness of breath and swollen ankles. Teach him to recognize and report these signs and symptoms.
• Check for breathing problems and light-headedness.
Interacting drug
• Antihypertensives
Possible effect
Additive hypotension. *Note:* This interaction is somewhat more significant with nifedipine.
Special considerations
• Periodically check blood pressure and pulse while the patient is lying down, sitting, and standing.
• Advise him to sit and stand slowly to avoid dizziness.
Interacting drug
• Digoxin
Possible effect
Digitalis toxicity from increased plasma digoxin levels. *Note:* This interaction is somewhat more significant with verapamil.
Special considerations
• Observe the patient for signs and symptoms of digitalis toxicity.
• Monitor plasma digoxin levels. Therapeutic levels range from 0.7 to 2.0 ng/ml.
• If necessary, suggest that the doctor reduce the digoxin dosage.
Continued

SPECIAL CONSIDERATIONS

Cardiovascular Drugs: Interactions Affecting Therapy
Continued

DIGITALIS GLYCOSIDES
All digitalis glycosides: for example, digitalis, digitoxin, digoxin

Interacting drug
• Potassium-wasting diuretics; for example, thiazide diuretics and loop diuretics
Possible effect
Digitalis toxicity from hypokalemia
Special considerations
• Monitor serum potassium levels.
• Check EKG readings for ST segment depression.
• Observe the patient for signs and symptoms of digitalis toxicity.
Interacting drug
• Thyroid hormones in very high doses
Possible effect
Reduced effectiveness of digitalis glycoside; mechanism unknown
Special considerations
• Monitor the patient for decreased response to digitalis glycoside. *Note:* A patient with a hyperthyroid condition may experience the same interaction.
Digoxin
Interacting drug
• Anticholinergics
Possible effect
Digoxin toxicity from increased intestinal absorption of digoxin
Special considerations
• Check the patient for signs and symptoms of digoxin toxicity.
Interacting drug
• Quinidine
Possible effect
Digoxin toxicity from altered digoxin distribution
Special considerations
• Monitor plasma digoxin levels. Therapeutic levels range from 0.7 to 2 ng/ml.
• Reduce the digoxin dosage, as ordered.
• Check the patient for signs and symptoms of digoxin toxicity.

POTASSIUM-SPARING DIURETICS
All potassium-sparing diuretics: amiloride, spironolactone, triamterene

Interacting drug
• Potassium supplements
Possible effect
Hyperkalemia from potassium retention
Special considerations
• Monitor serum potassium levels.
• Check EKG readings for widening of QRS complexes, tall T waves, and ventricular fibrillation.
• Observe the patient for other signs and symptoms of hyperkalemia.
• Instruct the patient to minimize intake of foods high in potassium.

GI Drugs: Interactions Affecting Therapy

Because antacids alter gastric pH, they can set the stage for various drug interactions. Cimetidine, an antiulcer drug, can slow drug metabolism and prolong other drugs' duration of action.

ALL ANTACIDS

Interacting drug
• All enteric-coated products, including some forms of aspirin; for example, Ecotrin
Possible effect
Premature drug dissolution in the stomach; antacids destroy enteric coating
Special considerations
• Administer drugs 1 hour apart.

ANTACIDS CONTAINING CALCIUM, MAGNESIUM, OR ALUMINUM
For example: Di-Gel*, Maalox Plus, Mylanta

Interacting drug
• Iron salts
Possible effect
• Decreased iron absorption from iron precipitation.
Special considerations
• Administer drugs 2 hours apart.
• Monitor the patient for decreased hematologic response to iron salt therapy.

*Not available in Canada

CIMETIDINE

Interacting drug
• All benzodiazepines (except lorazepam, oxazepam, and temazepam)
Possible effect
Excessive sedation from decreased metabolism of benzodiazepines
Special considerations
• Decrease benzodiazepine dosage, as ordered.
• Check the patient for unusual fatigue.
Interacting drug
• Theophylline
Possible effect
Theophylline toxicity from decreased theophylline metabolism
Special considerations
• Monitor plasma theophylline levels. Therapeutic levels range from 10 to 20 mcg/ml.
• Check the patient for signs and symptoms of theophylline toxicity.

Hormones: Interactions Affecting Therapy

Keep in mind that corticosteroids can make a patient susceptible to hypokalemia. If your patient's receiving a thiazide or loop diuretic while on corticosteroid therapy, be sure to continuously monitor serum potassium levels and check EKG readings periodically.

CORTICOSTEROIDS
All corticosteroids: for example, cortisone, dexamethasone, methylprednisolone, prednisone

Interacting drug
• Nonsteroidal anti-inflammatory drugs; for example, fenoprofen and ibuprofen
• Salicylates
Possible effect
GI ulcers from additive GI irritation
Special considerations
• Administer with food, milk, or antacids.
• Assess the patient for developing ulcers. Keep in mind that the anti-inflammatory drug may mask pain and other ulcer symptoms.
Interacting drug
• Digitalis glycosides
Possible effect
Digitalis toxicity from hypokalemia caused by corticosteroids
Special considerations
• Monitor serum potassium levels. Normal levels range from 3.8 to 5.0 mEq/liter.
• Observe the patient for signs and symptoms of digitalis toxicity.
• Encourage the patient to eat foods high in potassium, such as fruits and leafy green vegetables.
Interacting drug
• All potassium-wasting diuretics, especially thiazides and loop diuretics, or amphotericin B
Possible effect
Hypokalemia from additive effects
Special considerations
• Monitor serum potassium levels. Normal levels range from 3.8 to 5.0 mEq/liter.
• Periodically monitor the patient's EKG readings for signs of hypokalemia; for example, flat or inverted T waves, depressed ST segments, and widening of QRS complexes.
• Encourage the patient to eat foods high in potassium, such as fruits and leafy green vegetables.

Continued

SPECIAL CONSIDERATIONS

Hormones: Interactions Affecting Therapy
Continued

ORAL CONTRACEPTIVES

Interacting drug
● Barbiturates or rifampin
Possible effect
Reduced contraceptive effectiveness from increased metabolism of oral contraceptive
Special considerations
● Advise the patient to use an additional birth control method while taking barbiturates or rifampin, or ask the doctor to substitute one of the drugs with a noninteracting one.
Interacting drug
● Theophylline
Possible effect
Increased risk of theophylline toxicity because theophylline metabolism is inhibited by oral contraceptives

Special considerations
● Monitor plasma theophylline levels. Therapeutic levels range from 10 to 20 mcg/ml.
● Check the patient for signs and symptoms of theophylline toxicity: anorexia, nausea and vomiting, headache, tachycardia, dizziness, and restlessness.

THYROID HORMONES
All thyroid hormones: levothyroxine, liothyronine, liotrix, thyroglobulin, thyroid

Interacting drug
● Cholestyramine
● Colestipol
Possible effect
Decreased thyroid hormone effectiveness from decreased intestinal absorption of thyroid hormones
Special considerations
● Administer cholestyramine and colestipol at least 4 hours before or after a thyroid hormone.

Psychotherapeutic Drugs: Interactions Affecting Therapy

Tricyclic antidepressants (TCAs) have an anticholinergic effect. So, if you're administering a TCA with another anticholinergic drug (such as belladonna or propantheline), monitor your patient for blurred vision, drowsiness, constipation, urinary retention, and other signs and symptoms of excessive anticholinergic response.

Barbiturates speed the metabolism of many drugs.

Lithium can be toxic when given with indomethacin or a thiazide or loop diuretic. Stay alert for such adverse reactions as CNS depression, tremors, GI irritation, dizziness, headache, confusion, and mental dullness.

TRICYCLIC ANTIDEPRESSANTS (TCAs)
All tricyclic antidepressants: for example, amitriptyline, amoxapine, desipramine, doxepin, imipramine, maprotiline, nortriptyline, protriptyline, trimiparine.

Interacting drug
● Epinephrine or norepinephrine
Possible effect
Increased sympathomimetic effect from drug synergism
Special considerations
● Decrease the dosage of these sympathomimetic drugs, if ordered.
● Check the patient's history for cardiac problems.
Interacting drug
● Monitor for increased sympathomimetic effects, such as increased heart rate.
● Monitor blood pressure and pulse; report deviations from baseline.

BARBITURATES
All barbiturates: for example, amobarbital, butabarbital, pentobarbital, phenobarbital, secobarbital

Interacting drug
● Beta adrenergic blockers; for example, propranolol and metoprolol
Possible effect
Decreased beta adrenergic blocker effectiveness from increase in first-pass metabolism
Special considerations
● Monitor the patient for reduced effectiveness of beta adrenergic blocker. Consider the beta blocker to be effective if your patient's pulse rate doesn't increase after a position change from sitting to standing.
Interacting drug
● Corticosteroids, doxycycline, oral contraceptives, or quinidine
Continued

Psychotherapeutic Drugs: Interactions Affecting Therapy
Continued

BARBITURATES
Continued

Possible effect
Decreased effectiveness of the interacting drug from increased metabolism
Special considerations
• Increase dosage of the interacting drug, if ordered.
• Monitor the patient for decreased therapeutic effect.
• If the patient's using an oral contraceptive while receiving barbiturates, advise her to use an additional birth control method.
• If the patient's receiving quinidine with barbiturates, monitor plasma quinidine levels and check his EKG frequently.
Interacting drug
• Alcohol
Possible effect
Additive and synergistic CNS and respiratory depression
Special considerations
• Warn the patient to avoid alcohol, including over-the-counter drugs containing alcohol (for example, liquid cough and cold preparations).

LITHIUM

Interacting drug
• All potassium-wasting diuretics

(thiazides and loop diuretics) or indomethacin
Possible effect
Lithium toxicity from decreased lithium excretion
Special considerations
• Monitor plasma lithium levels. Toxic levels are above 1.5 mEq/liter.
• Monitor the patient for signs and symptoms of lithium toxicity.
• Warn the patient not to take any over-the-counter drugs (especially diuretics) unless the doctor or pharmacist approves.
• Before discharge, teach him to recognize signs and symptoms of lithium toxicity.
Interacting drug
• Methyldopa
Possible effect
Lithium toxicity from altered lithium distribution
Special considerations
• Monitor plasma lithium levels. Toxic levels are above 1.5 mEq/liter.
• Regularly assess the patient for adverse CNS effects.
• Monitor the patient for signs and symptoms of lithium toxicity.
• Before discharge, teach him to recognize signs and symptoms of lithium toxicity.

Continued

SPECIAL CONSIDERATIONS

Psychotherapeutic Drugs: Interactions Affecting Therapy
Continued

LITHIUM
Continued

Interacting drug
• Urinary alkalinizers; for example, antacids, carbonic anhydrase inhibitors
Possible effect
Decreased lithium effectiveness from hastened renal excretion of lithium
Special considerations
• Monitor plasma lithium levels and therapeutic response.
• Observe the patient for worsening of his psychiatric condition.
• Increase lithium dosage, if ordered.

MONOAMINE OXIDASE (M.A.O.) INHIBITORS
All MAO inhibitors: for example, isocarboxazid, phenelzine, procarbazine, tranylcypromine

Interacting drug
• Sympathomimetics; for example, amphetamines, norepinephrine, metaproterenol, and pseudoephedrine
Possible effect
Hypertension and other serious cardiovascular disorders from excessive catecholamine release

Special considerations
• Don't administer these drugs together.
• Advise the patient not to use over-the-counter preparations containing sympathomimetic drugs, such as diet pills, cold and allergy medicines, and nasal sprays. Tell him to check with the pharmacist before buying over-the-counter drugs.
Interacting drug
• Tricyclic antidepressants
Possible effect
Hypertension and other serious cardiovascular disorders
Special considerations
• Use this drug combination with caution.
• Monitor the patient's blood pressure and heart rate.
Interacting drug
• Levodopa
Possible effect
Levodopa toxicity from reduced levodopa metabolism
Special considerations
• Monitor the patient for signs and symptoms of levodopa toxicity, such as flushing, hypertension, and tachycardia.

INDEX

A

Abbreviations, 18
Acetaminophen toxicity, 156
Administration guidelines, 1-11
Administration problems, 5-6
Adverse reactions in elderly, 143-144
Air embolism, 117
Alcoholic solution, 25-26
Allergic reaction, 117
Allergic reaction precautions, 4
Allergic transfusion reaction, 135
Aminoglycoside interactions, 163-164
Amphotericin B interactions, 165-166
Antacid interactions, 178
Antiarrhythmic interactions, 173-174
Anticoagulant, oral, interactions, 169-170
Anticonvulsant interactions, 167-168
Antidiabetic, oral, interactions, 171-172
Antihypertensive interactions, 174-175
Anti-infective interactions, 163-166
Antineoplastic drugs, safe handling of, 148-149
Apothecary system, 13, 14

B

Barbiturate interactions, 181-182
Barbiturate toxicity, 156-157
Benzodiazepines, effects of, 155
Beta-adrenergic blocker interactions, 175-176

C

Calcium channel blocker interactions, 176
Calculations, 12-18
Capsule, administration of, 23-24
Carbamazepine interactions, 167
Cardiotonic glycoside toxicity, 157-158
Cardiovascular drug interactions, 173-177
Cartridge injection system, 66-67
Catheter embolism, 117
Central venous catheter, 100
Cephalosporin interactions, 164
Cimetidine interactions, 178
Circulatory overload, 116
Combining drugs in syringe, 68-70
Continuous drip (primary line infusion) method, 87, 90-92
Continuous subcutaneous insulin infuser, 79
Controlled drugs, schedule for, 10-11
Corticosteroid interactions, 179
Cream, 41
Cryoprecipitate, 137

D

Depressants, effects of, 155
Diabetic considerations for subcutaneous injections, 78
Dicumarol interactions, 169-170

Blood

Blood administration guidelines, 132-133
Blood components, 129-131
Blood contamination, 135
Buccal route, 30

INDEX

Digitalis glycoside interactions, 177
Drug abuse, 154-155
Drug interactions, 161-183
Drug laws, 7
Drug toxicities, 156-160

E

Ear drops, instillation of, 51-52
Elastomeric infusor, 105
Elderly patient, medications and, 141-144
Endotracheal medication administration, 63
Enema, 36, 38-39
Erythromycin interactions, 166
Extravasation, 98-99
Eye medication disk, 49-50
Eye medications, 47-50

F

Face mask, 61
Factor VIII concentrate, 137
Febrile transfusion reaction, 135
Five Rights, 1
Flow rate deviations, 119-120
Flow rates, calculation of, 21
Food, effect of, on drugs, 29

G

Gamma globulin, 137
Gastrostomy tube medication administration, 34-35
GI drug interactions, 178

H

Hemolytic transfusion reaction, 134

Heparin administration, 77
Heparin lock, 96
Home I.V. hyperalimentation complications, 127-128
Hormone interactions, 179-180
Household equivalents, 14
Hyperalimentation, 123-124
Hypertonic I.V. solutions, 121
Hypotonic I.V. solutions, 121

I

I.M. injections, 65, 80-86
I.M. injection sites, 80-81
Implantable drug delivery system, 105
Implanted infusion port, 101
Indwelling catheter, 100, 101
Infection at insertion site, 118
Infiltration, 116
Inhalation medications, 60-62
Injection routes, 64-65
In-line I.V. filters, 110
Inside-the-needle catheter, 111-112, 115
Intermittent (additive set) infusion, 87, 93-95, 96
Intraarterial infusion, 102-103
Intradermal injections, 64, 71-73
Intradermal injection sites, 71
Intrathecal injections, 104
IPPB therapy, 60
Isoniazid interactions, 166
Isotonic I.V. solutions, 121
I.V. bolus (push) injections, 87, 88-89
I.V. controllers, 150
I.V. fluid calculations, 16-17
I.V. fluids, 121-122

INDEX

I.V. injections, 65, 87-101
I.V. peripheral lines, 111-115
I.V. pumps, 150, 151
I.V. solution compatibility, 97
I.V. therapy, 19-21, 108-109
I.V. therapy complications, 116-118

L

Legal responsibility in drug administration, 7-9
Liquid oral medications, 25-28
Lithium interactions, 182-183
Lotion, 41

M

Mantoux (PPD) test for TB, 73
Medication syringe, 28
Meperidine interactions, 162-163
Metered-dose nebulizer, 57-58, 59
Metric system, 12, 14
Monoamine oxidase inhibitor interactions, 183
Mouth medications, 56

N

Narcotic interactions, 162
Narcotics, effects of, 154
Narcotic toxicity, 158-159
Nasal cannula, 61
Nasal inhaler, 58-59
Nasal medications, instillation of, 53-55
Nasogastric tube medication administration, 32-33
Nitroglycerin disk, 46
Nitroglycerin ointment, 43-44
Nonrebreather mask, 62

O

Ocusert, 105
Ointment, 36, 42
Opioid analgesic interactions, 162
Oral contraceptive interactions, 179-180
Oral medications, 23-29
Oropharyngeal inhalers, hand-held, 57-59
OROS (oral osmotic) drug delivery system, 105
Over-the-needle catheter, 111, 112, 114
Oxygen delivery systems, 61-62

P

Pain of I.M. injection, reducing, 86
Parenteral nutrition, 125-126
Partial rebreather mask, 62
Paste, 42
Pediatric medication administration, 138-140
Penicillin interactions, 165
Pennkinetic drug delivery system, 105
Phenobarbital interactions, 167
Phenytoin interactions, 168
Phlebitis, 116
Plasma, 130, 136
Plasma protein fraction, 131, 136
Plasma protein incompatibility, 135
Platelets, 130-131, 136
Potassium-sparing diuretic interactions, 177
Powder, 41

INDEX

Pregnant patient, drugs and, 146-147
Progestasert, 105
Proportions, setting up, 15
Propoxyphene interactions, 162
Prothrombin complex, 137
Psychotherapeutic drug interactions, 181-183

R

Reconstituted powders and tablets, 26
Rectal medications, 36-39
Red blood cells, 129
Retention enema, 38, 39

S

Salicylate interactions, 161-162
Salicylate toxicity, 159-160
Secondary I.V. line, 93-95
Sepsis, 118
Serum albumin, 131, 136
Spasmolytic toxicity, 160
Stimulants, effects of, 155
Stroke victim, medication administration and, 145
Subcutaneous injections, 64, 74-79
Subcutaneous injection sites, 74
Sublingual route, 30
Suppository, 36, 37
Suspension, 25
Syrup, 25

T

Tablets, administration of, 23-24
Tetracycline interactions, 165
Throat medications, 56
Thyroid hormone interactions, 180
Topical medications, 41-46
Transdermal medication application, 45
Transfusion reactions, 134-135
Tricyclic antidepressant interactions, 181
Tube medication administration, 31-35
Turbo-inhaler, 58, 59

V

Vaginal medications, 40
Venipuncture sites, 106-107
Venturi mask, 62
Volume-control I.V. set, 152-153

W

Warfarin interactions, 169-170
White blood cells, 129-130
Whole blood, 129
Winged infusion set, 111-112, 114

Z

Z-track method for injection, 85

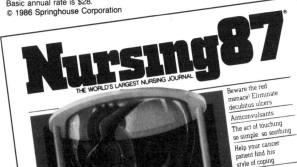